feeding your skin

Carla Oates has worked as a freelance writer for the last eight years. She writes a weekly DIY beauty column for the *Sunday Telegraph*, Australia, and is studying aromatherapy. Carla lives at Bondi Beach with her two children and one husband in a small apartment full of books, guitars, toys, window herbs and essential oils.

For Jeet and Otis, my beautiful babies

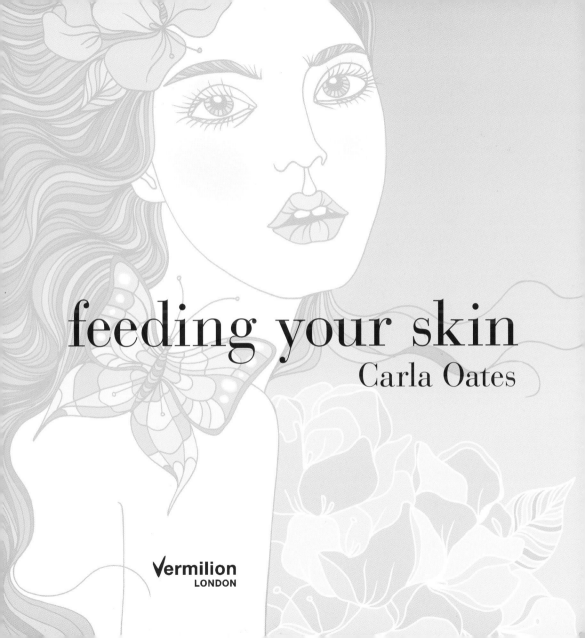

feeding your skin

Carla Oates

Vermilion
LONDON

1 3 5 7 9 10 8 6 4 2

Published in 2007 by Vermilion, an imprint of Ebury Publishing
A Random House Group company

First published in Australia by The Penguin Group in 2004

The Random House Group Limited Reg. No. 954009

Addresses for companies within the Random House Group can be found at
www.randomhouse.co.uk

A CIP catalogue record for this book is available from the British Library

The Random House Group Limited makes every effort to ensure that the papers used in our books are
made from trees that have been legally sourced from well-managed and credibly certified forests. Our paper
procurement policy can be found on www.randomhouse.co.uk

Cover and text design by Melissa Fraser
Author photograph by Simon Lekias

Printed and bound in Singapore by Tien Wah Press

ISBN 9780091922016

Copies are available at special rates for bulk orders. Contact the sales development team on
020 7840 8487 or visit
www.booksforpromotions.co.uk for more information.

To buy books by your favourite authors and register for offers, visit www.rbooks.co.uk

contents

body

acknowledgements

Big thanks to Julie Gibbs, Nicola Young, Melissa Fraser, my wonderful agent Pippa, amazing Grace, Angela, Curtis Brown, Linda Bates, Kevin Farrow, Gillian, Megan Mathews, Maree Mansour, Narelle Chenery and Carolyn Stubbin – for both your help and inspiration – and Anna Mason, Dad, Yasmin Sadikot, Ron Guba, Paul McNeil, Jay, Tom, Kerrie, Tory and Annette. And the biggest thanks of all to Davor and my mum for all their patience and support.

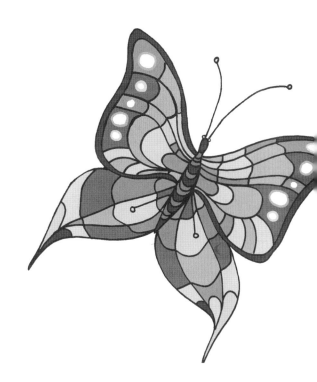

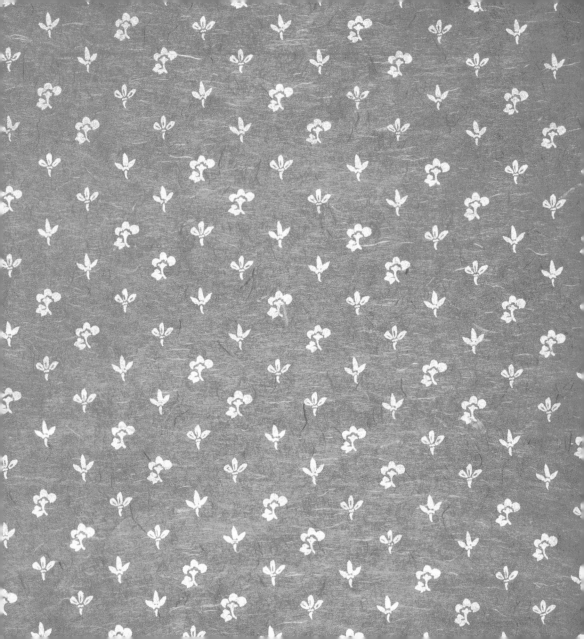

introduction

As small children, my sister and I delighted in concocting wild and wonderful lotions and potions. My mum tagged us the 'little witches' as we spent hours upon days furtively mixing her perfumes and cosmetics together with all sorts of odds and ends from the kitchen cupboard and clippings from the garden. Before long I had set up a healing clinic in the lounge room and employed our finest brews to help cure the imaginary skin conditions of any willing and brave patient (namely our parents). For my 'magic', we charged a small fortune.

So, as fate would have it, I find myself some twenty years later a beauty editor, both surrounded by and prescribing readers the gamut of ointments, creams, balms, unguents and make-up on the market. Only sadly, as I have come to discover, the ones in the fancy packaging contain very little magic at all. It seems that in our quest to look good and feel modern we have indiscriminately forsaken the knowledge handed down by generations of women – of nutritious homemade cosmetic recipes from the days when women successfully looked after their own skin. And at the mercy of sexy marketing campaigns we have entrusted big money-making companies with our health. Unfortunately, they are doing a very poor job.

Most of our favourite cosmetics are made with chemical solvents and synthetic additives – questionable substances that are directly absorbed into the body through the skin and over time may compromise our wellbeing. Even the pots of goo that trade under the 'green' banner are often full of undesirable ingredients. And this is not limited just to cosmetics for adults. We are exposed to these chemicals from the time our first nappy is changed. In fact, talcum powder, baby wipes, lotions and shampoos are some of the worst offenders. Unfortunately, most beauty products are not very beautiful at all and, as you know, neither are their price tags!

Life as a beauty editor puts you high up in the popularity stakes – you get sent loads of products – and at times I have felt like the local beauty pusher. My house has become the preferred venue for family lunches. The meal is usually followed by a casual utterance, 'Oh, by the way, I need a new moisturiser,' and we invariably end up in what my daughter calls 'mummy's product room'. Of late, I've been driving the 'go natural' bandwagon and placed an indefinite embargo on the product (poison!) room. I have 'progressed' back to childhood, concocting my own special chemical-free formulations for the skin and bottling them. I've been sticking pretty pictures on the bottles to seduce otherwise dubious punters, and have offered them as substitutes for mainstream brands.

To complement my packaged goods, I've been creating delicious and nutritious fresh food facials, cracking eggs into the hair, slathering avocado onto the skin, applying sugar scrubs to the body and waxing legs with sticky, buttery toffee. A wonderful rich, nutritious and tactile feast for the skin and hair, created using fresh and organic ingredients found in the fridge and bowl – without one harmful ingredient.

The responses from my guinea pigs have been very positive. Radiant skin and fun-filled afternoon cosmetic cook-ups have inspired comments like 'You should open a salon' or 'Write a book that I can keep alongside my favourite recipe books in the kitchen.' A cookbook for the skin? Brilliant!

This book is full of creative and delicious recipes and ideas to give you back the power of caring for your body. It is dedicated to anyone who wants to nurture his or her skin and body kindly and safely. It has become very apparent to me over the last couple of years that the women who anoint themselves with the purest of oils and botanical concoctions have the most radiant, succulent skin. This is enhanced by their holistic approach to beauty; they eat well, exercise and engage in activities that give them joy. After all, joy is a woman's best cosmetic! The other advantage of looking after yourself holistically is that you are contributing to a happier and healthier environment – only pure, unadulterated ingredients will be washed into our precious seas.

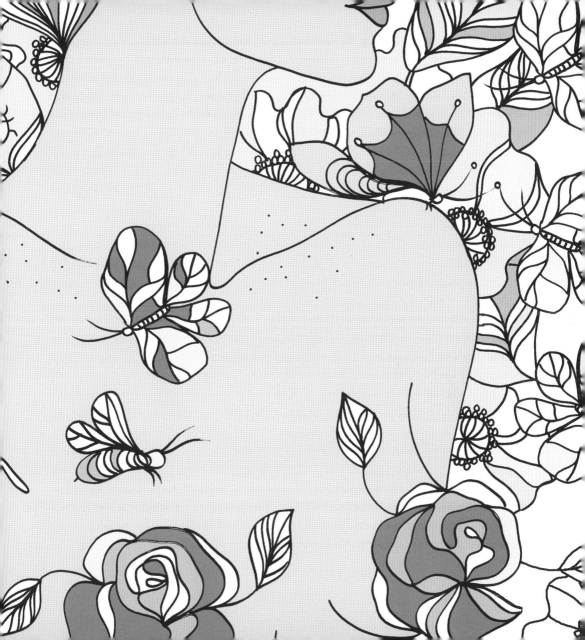

The recipes in this book come from myriad sources, some inspired by kitchen alchemists who have gone before me, some time-honoured remedies from ancient cultures including the wonderful world of Ayurvedic beauty. Others come from the inspiring people I have met on my journey – natural health practitioners who have generously and lovingly dedicated themselves to educating individuals on how to empower themselves. The rest come from me, experimenting for hours on end in the kitchen, a creative adventure of sorts that has not only altered the way I look after my skin, but the way I choose to live my life. Enjoy!

inner beauty

While the recipes in this book will promote healthy and radiant skin, you should remember that topical treatments work best alongside a diet rich in enzymes and other proteins, vitamins, essential fatty acids, minerals and anti-oxidants. I am forever telling my friends who complain about skin problems to spend their money on a naturopath rather than a beautician. The skin, hair and nails are the last stop for essential nutrients (which arrive at the most important organs first), so it's of the utmost importance to maintain a balanced diet and to consult a naturopath to check that you are assimilating nutrients properly. They will also work with you to ensure your body is eliminating toxins efficiently through the liver and kidneys, so all the impurities don't flood through your skin and cause skin conditions. Premature ageing of the skin can also be related to sun damage, stress, hormonal changes, too much sugar and refined foods, pollution, lack of exercise, and the use of harsh skincare products, so where possible avoid these things.

Confidence and inner peace give your face a radiance that cannot be replicated by make-up, as disturbances of the skin may reflect an emotional world out of balance. For peace of mind, it's important to deal with pent-up feelings. Talk to a therapist, do yoga and learn to meditate and be calm. Engage in activities you enjoy, and surround yourself with positive people who make you feel accepted and loved. Diminished levels of stress are guaranteed to bring about an improvement in your complexion, even without any special treatments.

So pull your shoulders back, drink lots of water, feed your skin, exercise and, most importantly, have lots of fun!

skin types

There is a generally accepted method of skin classification according to the balance of water and sebum in the tissues. Each category represents a state of imbalance.

5

normal is rare unless you're very young. It is soft, smooth, finely textured, supple and balanced in both oil and moisture content. It has no enlarged pores, wrinkles or blemishes and is firm and resilient.

oily has a coarser texture, with obvious enlarged pores. The skin may look sallow or dingy and is prone to acne, blackheads and infection. It's greasy as a result of over-production of sebum, which can be caused by a number of factors including heredity, bad diet, metabolic disorders, hormonal imbalances, insufficient skin hygiene or harsh preparations that strip the oil from the skin.

dry is usually delicate and fine-textured, with no obvious pores, and has a predisposition to facial lines and wrinkles. It lacks moisture or fat due to inadequate production by the sebaceous glands and an inability to trap surface moisture. Often it feels tight, parched and flaky.

combination is a mixture of two or more skin types, often dry patches with oily patches on the T-zones, where the sebaceous glands are most prevalent: the forehead, nose and chin. Each area is best treated according to its needs. For example, two types of mask should be prepared, one for each skin type.

introduction

sensitive is fine-textured and translucent, and often prone to lines and small surface veins. It can suffer redness and irritation when exposed to allergens in the air and to products such as perfume, lanolin and pollen. It is often more susceptible to eczema and dermatitis. People with this skin type are often very sensitive and finely tuned both physically and emotionally.

dehydrated is lacking in water, quickly wrinkled, drawn and often cold. Lack of water in the tissues can be caused by insufficient fluid intake, poor lymphatic function, dieting, climatic conditions, central heating or air-conditioning, or lack of sebum. Both dry and oily skins can become dehydrated.

mature or ageing is prone to dryness and dehydration, as it lacks oil and moisture, and to wrinkles and lines. The skin becomes flaccid, sags (with underlying fat-shrinkage and skin-loosening) and looks dull. Growths and pigmentation occur, and small capillaries appear.

acneous suffers from acne, a disease of the sebaceous glands and hair follicles. An excess of sebum is produced and clogs the pores, forming blackheads. The pressure of this sebum in the connective tissue increases, and creates inflammations, abscesses or pimples.

broken capillaries appears as small, dilated, winding, bright red blood vessels on the cheeks, around the nose and sometimes on the chin. It occurs as a result of poor elasticity of the capillary wall and gives the appearance of diffuse or local redness. It is aggravated by extremes of temperature, by excessively hot or cold water, nervous or digestive disorders, poor nutrition, saunas, exercise, drinking very hot liquids, spicy foods, blushing, smoking, alcohol, and aggressive scrubs and alcohol-based toners.

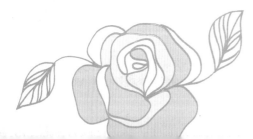

where
to
begin

the essential ingredients

You don't need the lore of a scientist to create radical skincare when the latest buzz ingredients are found in the most humble of foods. Fruit, flowers, veggies, herbs, dairy foods, beans, nuts and flours are rich in vitamins, minerals, fruit acids, enzymes, amino acids, alpha-hydroxy acids (AHAs), fatty acids, anti-oxidants, carbohydrates and proteins, providing you with all the active ingredients you need to create luxurious and sophisticated skincare.

Creating your own cosmetics may be a little time consuming, but if you dedicate a day every so often to replenishing your supplies, it can evolve into a lavish beauty ritual, inspiring you to take time out and nurture your body in a truly holistic way. Gather a group of friends and make a day of cosmetic cooking. That way you can share the costs and time and swap your delicious recipes. The recipes in this book are easy and cost very little, putting beauty and wellbeing within every goddess's reach.

buying ingredients

Some of the ingredients used in my recipes are more readily available than others. Dried herbs and roots can be purchased at the supermarket or from a health food shop. Floral waters and clays can be bought at a health food shop or chemist, or from a supplier. Essential oils can be found in many retail shops, but your local health food store or chemist, or a supplier, may be your best bet. To ensure that you are buying the pure distilled essences and not dubious chemical concoctions, look for the botanical name on the bottle and buy from a reputable, well-established company that specialises in essential oils. See page 165 for suppliers.

Opt for organic produce where possible. That way you can ensure your preparations are free of synthetic chemicals. Many mainstream supermarkets now sell organic produce.

hygiene & sterilisation

Good hygiene is an integral part of being a successful home cosmetician. Preparations contaminated with bacteria or mould can be harmful to the skin, especially when it is broken or cracked.

To keep your cosmetics as pure and safe as possible follow these tips.

- Tie your hair back if it's long.
- Wear an apron.
- Wash your hands well, before and during preparation.
- Keep towels handy to dry your hands.
- Ensure your utensils are clean.
- Clean your chopping boards with salt before you begin.

To sterilise glass or plastic containers, put them in boiling water for 20 minutes, then leave them to dry completely, away from pollutants and contaminants. Make sure the water used in your recipes is as pure as possible. If you use tap water, filter and boil it first.

your tools

You will need some basic tools, most of which you will already have in your kitchen. It is wise to keep some utensils separate from your cooking tools. Wooden spoons, for example, absorb flavours and smells – you don't want to end up with tea-tree-flavoured pancakes! Some substances like beeswax are also difficult to clean off surfaces. Here are some tools you might not already have.

- rubber spatulas
- measuring cups and spoons
- heat-resistant glass mixing bowls (Pyrex bowls are ideal)
- coffee filter papers
- mortar and pestle
- electric coffee grinder
- spray bottles
- pump bottles
- double boiler (bain-marie) or small saucepan with a Pyrex glass bowl that fits inside
- sensitive weighing scales (dieters' scales are inexpensive)
- glass dropper (for measuring essential oils and other small quantities)
- muslin (buy a metre-long piece and cut it into smaller square pieces)
- small and large funnels
- small battery-operated mixing wand
- two kitchen thermometers

Make sure that all your utensils are sterilised in boiling water, and do not use metal bowls or spoons, as they oxidise with fruit and vegetable juices and clay.

allergies

Although natural ingredients are less likely to cause an allergic reaction, it is possible they will. If a reaction occurs, wash the substance off your skin immediately. If it's an essential oil, remove it with a fatty oil, like olive or sweet almond oil. To test for allergens, do a patch test by applying one of the ingredients to a plaster and attaching it firmly to the soft skin just inside your elbow. Leave it on for 24 hours and check for any reaction. If you have particularly sensitive skin it may be worth carrying out patch tests before applying your preparations to the face. To test essential oils, add 1 drop to 1 teaspoon of vegetable oil and massage a little on the inside of your elbow. Cover with a plaster and leave for 24 hours. If there is no reaction, redness, soreness or itchiness, the ingredient is fine to use in your preparations.

vegetable oils, fats & waxes

Pure vegetable oils, fats and waxes are extracted from the seeds, kernels, nuts and other parts of plants. They are used widely in cosmetics to soften, smooth and moisturise skin and hair, and protect them from moisture loss. They're rich in essential fatty acids, anti-oxidants, vitamins and minerals, and provide effective, complementary bases for essential oils. Vegetable oils are best extracted without heat (which destroys many of their nutritive qualities) so opt for unrefined, cold-pressed varieties. Most cold-pressed oils will last up to 9 months in the fridge – at cold temperatures they tend to go cloudy, a good sign that they're unrefined. When buying sesame oil make sure it's the unrefined kind, not the dark-coloured oil used in Asian cooking!

clays

Argiletz (French) clays are cleansing, detoxifying, drawing, exfoliating, healing, soothing, toning and rejuvenating, and can be incorporated into cleansers, scrubs, masks, body powders, scalp treatments and bath preparations. They are available in five different colours, each offering properties suitable for a particular skin type. The depth at which active clays are extracted from the earth affects their active mineral content, colour and use. Green clay is the most absorbent and suited to acneous, oily and neglected skin; pink is purifying and toning and suitable for all skin types; red helps treat sensitive skin and broken capillaries; white is the gentlest, soothing, softening and suitable for all skin types; and yellow is recommended for restoring tired and neglected skin of all types.

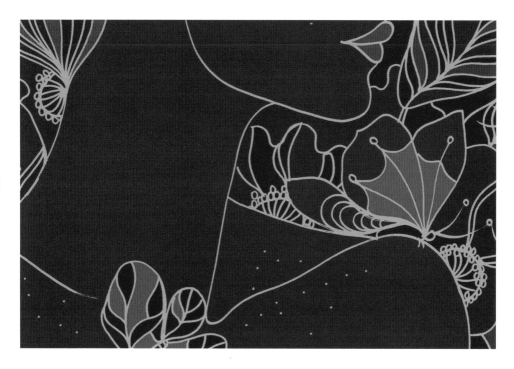

floral waters

Floral waters are also known as waters of distillation, or hydrosols. They are the by-product of essential oil distillation. They help hydrate, tone, soothe, heal and freshen the skin and are wonderful in cosmetic preparations. It is important to buy the authentic waters. For the recipes in this book I have used chamomile water, lavender water, orange blossom water, rosewater and jasmine water. See page 159 for skin types these floral waters are suited to.

aromatherapy

Essential oils work wonderfully in skincare, providing all the elements required for healthy skin function. Their rejuvenating, antiseptic and tonic properties can help prevent or clear skin congestion and stimulate the generation of new cells. Because of their quite small molecular size, they penetrate deep into the dermis and beyond into the bloodstream to provide further therapeutic effects. They also help balance our emotions through their wondrous scent. In fact their emotional resonance is so powerful, it's very important that you like the scent of the oil for it to work effectively.

Essential oils can be incorporated into cleansers, creams, lotions, ointments, gels, toilette waters and perfumes. You can use them at 1 per cent dilution (around 20 drops in 5 tablespoons of a preparation). Essential oils alone or combined make beautiful therapeutic perfumes. The benefits of essential oils are that they:

- are highly antiseptic
- help speed up removal of old skin cells and promote growth of new ones
- improve muscle tone and blood circulation
- help eliminate waste
- reduce inflammation
- regulate sebum production, and
- reduce the impact of emotional stress.

precautions

Essential oils are highly concentrated forms of plant energy and can be harmful if not used properly; 1 drop of essential oil is said to have the therapeutic value of about 6 litres of herbal infusion. Do not take essential oils internally (unless prescribed by a practitioner) and keep them far away from children. Do not apply pure essential oils directly onto the skin and never exceed the recommended dose.

pregnancy

Many aromatherapists recommend that women avoid the use of some essential oils during pregnancy, especially in the first 3 months. You should always consult a qualified aromatherapist before using any aromatherapy products, even those you have made at home.

oil for babies

It is important to use a very low dilution on babies, due to their sensitive skin and small body size. You should only use very safe oils such as German and Roman chamomile, lavender, mandarin, tangerine and neroli. Use a 0.5 per cent dilution (1 drop in 2 teaspoons of base oil).

photosensitivity

Certain essential oils can render the skin photosensitive, making it more prone to burning when exposed to ultraviolet light. These are: angelica root, bergamot, bitter orange, cold-pressed lime, grapefruit and lemon. It's best to avoid the sunlight for at least 12 hours after applying any of these oils, although they are fine in cleansers if washed off thoroughly.

skin irritations

These oils may cause irritation to sensitive skin: basil, cinnamon leaf and bark, clove bud, lemon, lemongrass, tea-tree and thyme. Sensitivity varies from person to person and oil to oil.

pure essential oil compositions

Here are some suggestions for essential oil combinations for particular skin types. These quantities can be added to 5 tablespoons of base oil.

normal 10 drops lavender, 6 geranium, 4 ylang-ylang

oily 8 drops sandalwood, 6 lemon, 6 lavender

dry 8 drops sandalwood, 6 geranium, 6 rose

combination 10 drops lavender, 6 geranium, 4 orange

sensitive 6 drops chamomile, 4 rose, 2 neroli

dehydrated 10 drops rose, 8 sandalwood, 2 patchouli

mature 8 drops neroli, 6 frankincense, 6 ylang-ylang

acneous 10 drops lemon, 10 cypress, 5 lavender

devitalised 10 drops geranium, 6 rose, 4 cypress

broken capillaries 8 drops rose, 6 chamomile, 6 cypress

aromatherapy

preserving your creations

Anti-microbial preservatives reduce the growth of bacteria and fungi in your preparations. Instead of using parabens and the formaldehyde-based preservatives found in a lot of commercial cosmetics, look out for healthier alternatives like grapefruit seed extract (also known as citrus seed extract or citricidal), an anti-microbial and fungicidal – add at 0.5-3 per cent to water or herbal infusion. To help prevent your vegetable and nut oils from oxidising add anti-oxidants: 1-5 per cent vitamin E (tocopherol) oil to your total oil content, which is 1-5 ml per 100 ml. Or amiox (rosemary extract or herbalox) at 0.1-0.5 per cent which is approximately 2-10 drops every 100 ml.

the skin's little darlings

anti-oxidants fight free radicals. Vibrantly coloured fruits, veggies and herbs are rich in carotenoids, such as lutein, beta-carotene, lycopene and alpha-lipoeic acid, all powerful anti-oxidants. The denser the colour, it seems, the higher the anti-oxidant content. Vibrant orange foods like apricots, calendula, carrots, mangoes, oranges, papaya, pumpkin, rockmelon, rosehip and sweet potato are rich in the major anti-oxidant beta-carotene. Brilliant red and pink foods like tomatoes, watermelon and pink grapefruit are wonderful sources of lycopene. Green and black tea are also rich in anti-oxidants.

AHAs (alpha-hydroxy acids) and fruit enzymes accelerate the skin's natural shedding process by dissolving the dead, flaking skin of the epidermis (outer layer) and exposing the newer and smoother skin underneath.

fatty acids plump up the skin cells, helping them retain moisture, and restore the barrier function of the skin.

vitamin A helps improve the skin's elasticity and thickness, reduces the signs of photo-ageing and is also very healing for acneous skin. It is found in apple, carrot seed oil, cod liver, dandelion, egg yolks, milk, orange, tomato and yoghurt.

vitamin C is a potent anti-oxidant that helps heal wounds, stimulate collagen and promote elastin, therefore improving skin's elasticity and tone and diminishing the appearance of fine lines and wrinkles. It also fights free radicals – triggered by sun exposure, pollution or stress – which can damage the skin. It's found in vegetables, herbs, grains and citrus fruits.

vitamin E is an anti-oxidant and anti-inflammatory emollient that helps fight free radicals, soothes and smooths the skin, and aids in tissue healing. It's found naturally in vegetables, oils, nuts, seeds, whole grains, wheat flour and dairy products. Make sure you buy vitamin E in its natural form, tocopherol.

longevity of cosmetics

- All emulsions will last up to 6 months, especially if kept refrigerated.
- All dry scrubs, if kept dry, will last up to 6 months, especially if kept refrigerated.
- Any formulations containing alcohol will last up to 1 year.
- Treatment oils with amiox or vitamin E added should last between 6 and 9 months.
- Balms should last up to 6 months, especially if kept refrigerated.
- Any herbal infusion or water-based products will last up to 3 days in the fridge without citrus seed extract.
- Fresh masks will last 1-2 days.

basic recipes

These recipes provide the basic methods you will need to make the preparations in the Face and Body sections. You can also use them as a starting point for creating your own recipes.

herbal preparations

Dried herbs in dry preparations will keep, but once they are in the form of a decoction or infusion, they will only last a couple of days. Add up to 80 ml vodka to the recipes below to prevent them from spoiling.

When making these preparations, avoid using metal pots and containers, as they may react with the herb. Instead, use Pyrex, enamel or china vessels. To extract the active ingredients from the herbs, it's a good idea to pummel them first using a mortar and pestle.

infusions

Herbal infusions make wonderful remedial face washes and toners and can be incorporated into almost any preparation. The softer, more delicate parts of the plant (the flowers and leaves) are used. See page 159 for herbs to suit your skin type.

2 teaspoons dried herb or 4 teaspoons fresh herb, finely chopped
250 ml boiling water

1 Place the herb in a heat-resistant pitcher or bowl. Cover the herb with the boiling water and leave to steep for at least 15 minutes, covering the pot to prevent the loss of volatile elements through evaporation.
2 Strain the infusion.

where to begin

decoctions

To make a decoction, the herb is boiled gently in water to extract the active ingredients. The harder parts of the plant, like the roots, rhizomes, bark, seeds and berries, are usually treated in this way. The resultant decoction can be used in the same way as an infusion.

375 ml water
2 teaspoons dried or 4 teaspoons chopped or crushed fresh herb

1 Put the water in a saucepan with the herbs and bring to the boil. Cover tightly and simmer gently for 25 minutes.
2 Strain and filter if necessary.

vinegars

Herbal vinegars can be used as skin tonics, wound solutions, body splashes, deodorants, hair rinses and bath additives. Apple cider vinegar provides an ideal base.

1 Fill a jar with chopped fresh herbs or half-fill a jar with dried herbs, and pour in enough apple cider vinegar to fill the jar. Secure the lid.
2 Leave the jar in a warm, protected place for 2 weeks and shake the bottle twice daily.
3 Strain and filter, then bottle and store in a cool place, preferably the fridge.

tinctures

Herbal tinctures, often referred to as 'mother tinctures', are stronger and more concentrated than infusions or decoctions and have a much longer shelf life. The minimum concentration of alcohol needed for preservation is 40 per cent of a preparation. You need to use an alcohol that is at least 60 per cent proof. Vodka is around this amount. Because alcohol is an excellent solvent for plant materials, tinctures have potent remedial and healing qualities.

30 g dried herb
250 ml vodka

1 Place the herb in a jar and pour over the vodka.
2 Seal the jar, leave in a cool place and shake twice daily for 2 weeks.
3 Strain and filter through muslin (cheesecloth) and then through coffee filter paper.
4 Store in a dark glass bottle.

infused oils

A herbal infused oil works well in creams, ointments, and massage and bath oils. To make, you will need fresh herbs and a light, almost odourless, cold-pressed vegetable oil such as jojoba, sweet almond or apricot kernel oil.

1 Fill a jar with freshly chopped herbs and/or flowers. If only using herbs, half-fill the jar.
2 Cover the herbs with vegetable oil until the jar is full.
3 Seal the jar, leave in a warm place for 2 weeks (not in direct sunlight or the oil will become rancid) and shake twice daily. Delicate flowers like jasmine and honeysuckle decompose quickly, so it's important to replace them daily.
4 Strain through muslin (cheesecloth). Pour into a jar and store in the fridge.
5 After a few days, carefully decant the oil into a glass bottle, leaving the sediment behind. Refrigerate.

ointments & balms

Ointments, balms and salves are made from oils, waxes and fats and have no water content. They are thick and buttery, combine well with herbs and essential oils, and are used to help heal dry, irritated skin. They provide the skin with more protection than normal moisturisers, as they stay on the surface of the skin longer, making them ideal for treating chapped lips and nappy rash (but they should not be left on excessively oily skin). Jars of ointment will keep for months in the refrigerator, and make superb gifts.

Beeswax, cocoa butter, vegetable oils and shea butter are the basic ingredients. Sweet almond oil, apricot oil and jojoba oil are ideal vegetable oils, as they remain relatively stable when heated.

3–5 tablespoons vegetable oil
15 g beeswax
10 g cocoa butter

ointment method 1 – using herbs
1 Generously cover 30–50 g of dried or 90–150 g of fresh herb with the oil and warm gently in a bain-marie until the herb loses its normal colour.
2 Strain and allow to cool.
3 Melt the beeswax and cocoa butter in a bain-marie over low heat.
4 Remove from the heat and add the herbal oil, mixing well.
5 Pour into glass jars.

ointment method 2 – using herbal tinctures
1 Melt the vegetable oil, beeswax and cocoa butter together in a bain-marie.
2 Add 2 teaspoons of a herbal tincture, mixing thoroughly.
3 Pour into glass jars.

ointment method 3 – using finely ground dried herb

1 Melt the oil, beeswax and cocoa butter in a bain-marie.
2 Stir in 1–3 tablespoons of finely ground dried herb and simmer for 20 minutes.
3 Strain through muslin (cheesecloth) then coffee filter paper and pour into glass jars.

ointment method 4 – using herbal infused oil

1 Melt the beeswax and cocoa butter with the infused oil (instead of the vegetable oil) in a bain-marie and mix thoroughly.
2 Pour into glass jars.

mayonnaises

A mayonnaise made from fresh organic eggs, cold-pressed vegetable oils and aromatic essential oils is a sumptuous feast for thirsty skin and hair. It makes an easy, inexpensive, luxurious and convenient face and body cleanser, moisturiser, bath cream or hair treatment. You can use any high-quality oil, although you should choose one to suit your skin type (page 159). A batch will last for 2–3 weeks in the fridge. Measure your drops of essential oil with a plastic pipette.

1 egg yolk
250 ml cold-pressed vegetable oil
1 teaspoon honey
½ teaspoon apple cider vinegar
20 drops essential oil (optional – vanilla oil is lovely in this recipe)

1 Beat the egg yolk in a blender.
2 Slowly pour in the vegetable oil and continue mixing until the noise of the blender changes – a sign the mixture is getting thicker.
3 Slowly add the remaining ingredients, in order, mixing until well combined.

plant gels

Gel formulations are very hydrating and soothing. They make good oil-free cleansers, moisturisers and masks, eye treatments and hair gels, and are particularly useful in the warmer months when skin becomes greasier. Gels can be made from myriad foods; those most commonly used are linseeds, pectin (from citrus peel), guar gum, xanthan gum, arrowroot, Irish moss, marshmallow root, agar-agar and tapioca. Aloe vera gel can also make a suitable gel base.

Plant gels are made by adding water to pectin, guar or xanthan gum. They will only last a couple of days in the fridge, although adding a preservative like grapefruit seed extract will increase their longevity.

basic plant gel

This gel can be used as a moisturiser, eye gel or mask.

5 tablespoons purified water or floral water
¼–3 teaspoons powdered pectin or xanthan gum (depending on the desired consistency)
10 drops essential oil

1 Warm the water or floral water over a medium heat (do not boil) then remove from heat.
2 Sprinkle the powdered gum slowly into the water or floral water and whisk until the desired consistency is reached.
3 To make the gel smooth, push it through a strainer. If it is too thick for your liking, add more water.
4 Add the essential oil and mix well.

linseed gel

Linseed gel is emollient and very soothing. It is an excellent first aid gel for all manner of bruises, sprains, swellings, inflammations and burns. It also makes an impressive soothing, calming and plumping mask.

2 tablespoons linseeds
250 ml boiling water or herbal infusion

1 Simmer the linseeds in the boiling water or herbal infusion until a gel forms.
2 Strain the seeds from the gel, retaining the water or herbal infusion. Dilute with the strained water or herbal infusion if a thinner consistency is desired.

emulsions

Oil and water don't mix. However, with the use of an emulsifier, they can be bound together to form milky or creamy mixtures called 'emulsions'. Mayonnaise is an example of an emulsion and the ingredient (the emulsifier) that binds oil and vinegar together in a consistent form is the egg yolk. Without an emulsifier, you'd end up with a mixture similar to salad dressing, where the vinegar sits buoyantly on top of the oil. Most commercial cleansers and moisturisers are emulsions, and emulsions are the most complex preparations in this book. The secret? It's all in the way you mix. Depending on what goes together and how it is mixed, you can end up with either an omelette or a soufflé! But with practice, it becomes very easy and you can make a year's supply of face cream within an hour.

There are two types of emulsion. The first is an oil-in-water emulsion, which contains mostly water. Emulsions in this group include cleansing milks, cleansing creams, face creams and body lotions. The second type is a water-in-oil emulsion, which contains mostly oil. These emulsions feel thicker and greasier on the skin and include cold creams, ointments and barrier creams.

When an emulsion is made, two phases – the oil phase and the water phase – are required. In both phases, the ingredients are heated. Once the desired temperature is reached, the products of the two phases are combined to form the emulsion.

You can add your desired combination of pure essential oils, infused oils, cold-pressed vegetable oils, floral waters, herbal infusions and herbal tinctures. See page 159 for ingredients to suit your skin type. Measure your drops of essential oils and preservatives with plastic pipettes.

For 100 g

oil phase
6-8 g plant-derived emulsifying wax (plus other solid fats, as given in individual recipes)
15 ml vegetable oil or infused oil
4 drops rosemary leaf extract

water phase
75 ml purified or demineralised water
1 teaspoon vegetable glycerine

third phase
20 drops essential oil suited to your skin type (see pages 15 and 159)

1 Melt the waxes (and other solid fats) and the vegetable or infused oil (unless the oil is high in fatty acids, such as avocado, evening primrose, linseed or rosehip oil, which deteriorate if exposed to high heat for too long, in which case it should be added at stage 2) together in a bain-marie over a medium heat, stirring occasionally until well mixed.
2 Remove from the heat and add any vegetable oils high in fatty acids and the rosemary leaf extract to the heated oils and waxes. At 65°C, your mix is ready for the water phase.
3 Heat the combined water and glycerine to 65°C then slowly add to the oil phase over a low

heat, mixing continuously using a small hand-held mixing wand.

4   Remove from heat. The emulsion will be very watery in consistency and look milky. Continue mixing (oil-in-water emulsions can separate, so stir briskly) for a short time (about 20 seconds at the most). If the mixture does separate, simply remix it. Keep stirring by hand until the mixture starts to thicken and cool. Water-in-oil emulsions need to be stirred slowly and steadily.

5   When the emulsion has cooled a little, add the essential oils (third phase).

6   Pour into small jars.

aromatherapy ointments & balms

Aromatherapy ointments and balms can be used as massage balms, healing ointments or perfume balms.

15 g beeswax

10 g cocoa butter

3–5 tablespoons cold-pressed vegetable oil (and/or shea butter)

20–80 drops essential oil (add more or less depending on desired strength)

1   Melt the beeswax and cocoa butter with the vegetable oil or shea butter in a bain-marie, then remove from heat.

2   When the mixture starts to cool, add the essential oils and mix thoroughly.

3   Pour into glass jars.

face

cleansers

I must confess that a few honest splashes of water over a night-out's worth of dirt and make-up have often left me kidding myself that I've cleaned my face. But skin is too smart for such play. By the following morning, without fail, my skin has retaliated with a generous outburst of spots. As tempting as it may be, cleansing should never be a slapdash affair. It is the first and most important step in your skincare ritual, gently removing excess oil, make-up, pollution, grit and grime accumulated during the day. It also helps loosen dead skin cells, dislodge blackheads and clean out pores. Poorly cleansed skin leaves oil glands congested with dirt and cellular waste – the perfect environment for unwanted breakouts.

Most commercial cleansers contain surfactants like sodium lauryl sulfate, which strip the skin of its natural oils and upset its pH. This can often irritate the skin and send oil glands into overdrive, making oily skin even slicker. Soapy suds and big foamy bubbles may be impressive, but they do not clean better than other, milder cleansers; they just indicate a harsh product. Soap is harsh, leaves skin feeling parched, tight and uncomfortable, and is best avoided.

Gently press the face with a warm, damp soft cloth to help loosen clogged pores and soften surface cells. Apply your cleanser using sparklingly clean hands, a cotton cloth or organic cotton wool balls, depending on the cleanser used. If using your hands, massage the cleanser into

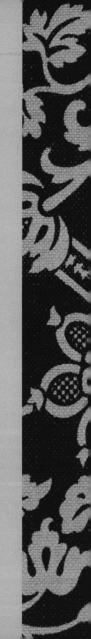

the face and neck using an upward circular motion, pressing along the main meridians of the face and neck and behind the ears. This facilitates the flow of oxygen-carrying blood to the face, enhancing the tone and texture of the complexion. To remove, always use a cotton cloth or flannel – splashing water from cupped hands will not lift surface grime. Muslin (cheesecloth) wash cloths are my favourite medium for removing cleansers, as they gently exfoliate the skin and wipe away the residue. Take your time, and as you wash away your cleanser, imagine the day's worries flowing steadily down the sink. When finished, rinse your cloth thoroughly and hang to dry. Replace every two days with a fresh, clean cloth. Sometimes it's a good idea to cleanse twice: once to remove surface dirt and make-up and a second time to get the skin really clean.

As the seasons change, so too will your cleanser requirements. In colder months, you may need a richer, more nourishing cleanser than in summer, when skin produces more oil. During a stressful patch your skin may become sensitive or dehydrated and require a different cleanser to cater for and help remedy the imbalance.

Use your cleanser twice daily: once lightly in the morning to remove waste the skin has expelled overnight and once in the evening to wash away the day's collection of dirt.

fresh milk & cream cleansers

Splash fatty, silky milk or smooth yoghurt over your face for a fine complexion. Nature's own skin-softening elixirs, they are replete with acids, lipids and enzymes, which help remove dead skin cells, prevent blackheads and smooth the skin. The high fat content of milk promotes a finer complexion and soothes reddened, dry or irritated patches. For dry and mature skin use full-fat milk, soya milk or cream; for oily complexions, skimmed milk is ideal. Yoghurt and buttermilk work well for all skin types, especially oily and untoned, and goat's milk, buttermilk and soya milk are kind on the most sensitive skin. Fresh milk cleansers can be used alone or with herbs and essential oils. Store in an airtight bottle in the fridge for up to 1 week.

Apply with an organic cotton wool ball in upward, circular motions, then rinse with lots of tepid water and a clean cotton wool ball. I prefer to use a milk cleanser in the morning and something a little more rigorous in the evening.

rich maple & rose geranium cleanser

FOR MATURE SKIN

In the depths of winter, when your skin is feeling parched, this cream will cleanse and nourish the skin. Maple syrup has many similar curative properties to honey, while rose geranium has excellent regenerative properties and so is ideal for mature skin. It gives a fresh floral edge to the warm, caramel-like maple scent.

1–2 drops rose geranium essential oil
1 tablespoon maple syrup
3 tablespoons cream

Add the rose geranium oil and maple syrup to the cream and mix thoroughly.

lavender buttermilk cleanser

FOR ALL SKIN TYPES, ESPECIALLY OILY AND COMBINATION

This delightful cleanser will give your complexion a lovely glow. Buttermilk is an effective astringent and has a noticeably toning effect. It brightens the skin and helps even out tone and reduce pore size.

1–2 drops lavender essential oil
62 ml buttermilk or milk to suit your skin type

Drop the lavender oil into the buttermilk or milk, mix well and bottle.

honey cream cleanser

FOR ALL SKIN TYPES

This mildly astringent cleanser will cleanse, tone and smooth. It is especially useful for skin that needs a lift.

1 teaspoon honey
1 teaspoon natural yoghurt

1 In a small bowl, combine the honey and yoghurt (you may need to warm the honey first) thoroughly.
2 Apply to damp skin with hands, rinse thoroughly with a damp, tepid cloth three times and pat dry with a soft towel.

cleansing oils

Cleansing oils have been used in various cultures for centuries and are still very popular in the Middle East. Unrefined, cold-pressed vegetable and nut oils are superb skin cleansers. Unlike the mineral oils found in most commercial cleansers, they don't just sit on the skin, but dissolve impurities on the surface of the skin while feeding it with nutrients. As strange as it may sound, cleansing oily skin with oil is very effective. With the oil layered onto the skin, the sebaceous glands are tricked into thinking they have produced enough oil and don't make more. Light oils like jojoba, hazelnut, sweet almond and apricot kernel are ideal for oily skin.

Recommended base oils for all skin types are jojoba, sweet almond, apricot kernel, sesame, sunflower and grape seed. Small percentages of heavier oils like avocado and wheat germ can be added for drier, more mature skin. Apply a cleansing oil to a damp face and massage over face and neck, then remove with a damp face washer and lots of tepid water. Your oil cleanser will last up to 6 months in a cool dark place. Add the contents of 2 vitamin E capsules to help preserve. Follow with a toner.

queen bee oil cleanser

FOR ALL SKIN TYPES

A mix of honey and almond oil makes an excellent facial cleanser for lifting stubborn city grime.

½ teaspoon honey
½ teaspoon sweet almond oil

Mix the honey into the sweet almond oil (you may need to warm the honey first). Make fresh as needed.

panda eyes cleansing oil

FOR ALL SKIN TYPES

This is a gentle, sweetly scented oil cleanser, perfect for lifting make-up around the delicate eye area.

4 tablespoons sweet almond oil
1 tablespoon apricot kernel oil
1 teaspoon vitamin E oil
3 drops chamomile essential oil

Pour or drop all the oils into a bottle, then seal and shake vigorously.

miss priss cleansing oil

FOR ALL SKIN TYPES

This cleanser has good antimicrobial action and a beguiling and uplifting scent. I often use it in the evening, when my skin feels like it is carrying the weight of the world.

4 tablespoons sweet almond oil
1 tablespoon apricot kernel oil
1 teaspoon vitamin E oil
7 drops mandarin essential oil
6 drops sandalwood essential oil
5 drops lavender essential oil
2 drops lemon essential oil

Combine the oils thoroughly. Store in a well-sealed glass bottle.

citrus infused oil cleanser

My husband uses this after welding, building or gardening, when a lot of soot and dirt visits his complexion. The citrus peel is extremely cleansing and the oil will help shift impurities.

zest of 1 lemon
zest of 1 lime
zest of 1 orange
5 g beeswax
5 tablespoons sweet almond oil

1 Dry the citrus zest in a 120°C (250°F, Gas Mark 1) oven for 1 hour, then grind into a powder.
2 Melt the beeswax with the sweet almond oil in a bain-marie, add the zest and infuse for 30 minutes over a low heat.
3 Strain through coffee filter paper and bottle.
4 Shake well before each use.

oats cleansers

Oats are remarkably cleansing, healing, anti-inflammatory, softening and moisturising. They are also high in silica and therefore great for skin, nails and hair. For years, professionals have heralded oats as the healing grain, recommending them for irritated and sensitive skin. Keep a jar of fine oatmeal near your sink, in the shower and bath, and use to cleanse every inch of your body. Add a couple of drops of lavender essential oil to each container to make the oats fragrant. Wrap a handful of oats in a piece of muslin (cheesecloth) and use as a wash ball on babies' tender skin. They will love it!

almond milk or oat milk paste cleanser

FOR ALL SKIN TYPES

Soak almond meal or oatmeal overnight in a milk suited to your skin type (page 159) and use the mix to cleanse your face in the morning. Both combinations are very cleansing and hydrating, and will keep the skin blemish-free.

long-life emulsion cleansers

mandarin & ylang-ylang milk cleanser

FOR ALL SKIN TYPES

You can alter the essential oils for a light and divinely fragrant cleanser to suit your skin type (page 159).

oil phase
7 g plant-derived emulsifying wax
15 ml apricot kernel oil
5 drops rosemary leaf extract

water phase
80 ml purified water or floral water
14 drops grapefruit seed extract

third phase

12 drops mandarin essential oil

8 drops ylang-ylang essential oil

Follow the instructions for making an emulsion on page 24.

lady muck's honey & sandalwood cleansing cream

FOR MATURE AND VERY DRY SKIN

This rich, grounding cleansing cream is also ideal for tortured, parched winter skin.

oil phase

8 g plant-derived emulsifying wax

2 g cocoa butter

15 ml sweet almond oil

5 ml honey

6 drops rosemary leaf extract

water phase

70 ml rosewater or purified water

12 drops grapefruit seed extract

third phase

20 drops sandalwood essential oil

Follow the instructions for making an emulsion on page 24.

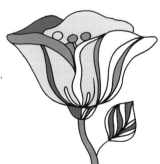

foaming cleansers

Castile soap is unlike other soaps, which often strip the skin of its natural oils. It is readily available at health food shops and offers a very gentle way to cleanse the face. You can adapt it by adding other ingredients to suit your skin type. Mixed with vegetable and nut oils, these cleansers produce a smooth, creamy non-drying lather. The essential oils make these cleansers beautifully fragrant and enhance their cleansing, soothing and antibacterial properties. These cleansers will last up to 6 months.

Apply a small amount to your fingertips, lather and apply to a damp face. Massage in upward circular motions. Remove with a cotton cloth and lots of tepid water.

castile cleanser

FOR ALL SKIN TYPES

In winter, when your skin is very dry, you may want to up the oil component to 1 tablespoon.

4½ tablespoons liquid Castile soap
2 teaspoons sweet almond or apricot kernel oil
20 drops essential oil suited to your skin type (page 159)

Pour or drop all the ingredients into a bottle and shake well.

soapwort cleanser

Soapwort is probably one of the gentlest ways to cleanse very sensitive skin. It contains natural saponins, which create an impressive lather.

1 tablespoon chopped and bruised soapwort root
375 ml water
1 teaspoon dried red clover or calendula flowers

1 Mix the herbs and water together and bring to the boil in a small saucepan.
2 Place over a low heat and simmer gently for 15 minutes.
3 Remove from heat, allow to cool, then strain and bottle. To thicken add a little citrus pectin or xanthan gum.
4 Use within 3-4 days or freeze in ice cube trays for later use.

geranium & clay cleanser

FOR OILY AND ACNEOUS SKIN

20 drops geranium essential oil
2 teaspoons jojoba oil
4 tablespoons liquid Castile soap
2 teaspoons green clay

1 Add the essential oil and jojoba oil to the Castile soap and mix well.
2 Mix in the clay well, smoothing out any clumps.

treatment cleanser

very dandy plum

FOR ANGRY, ACNEOUS SKIN

Juicy red plums are in season in the summer months, when oily and acneous skin are usually at their worst – perfect timing for cooking up this wonderful cleanser. Plums are astringent and benefit skin with a combination of large pores, blackheads and red, inflamed pimples. Dandelion leaves and roots boast vitamins A and C, both vital in treating acne.

2 plums, peeled, halved and stoned
375 ml water
2 teaspoons honey
1 teaspoon dried dandelion herb
1 teaspoon apple cider vinegar

1 Put all the ingredients in a small saucepan, bring to a boil and simmer over a low heat for 20 minutes.
2 Remove from the heat, allow to cool, then bottle.
3 Use cotton wool balls to wipe over the face then rinse well with tepid water. Use 3 times a week and make fresh each week or freeze a batch in ice-cube trays.

toners

Toners are refreshing elixirs applied to the skin after cleansing or mask-
ing to help remove or dissolve any residue. They are also used to help
stimulate circulation, restore the skin's acid mantle, hydrate and refine
the skin, and temporarily reduce pore size. Avoid alcohol-based toners,
which strip the skin of its natural oils, overstimulating the sebaceous
glands and making your skin far greasier than before. The ideal toner
should heal while correcting the skin's balance.

    Apply with a cotton wool ball after cleansing, in gentle, circular,
upward motions. Leave on and follow with a moisturiser or lotion to suit
your skin type.

aloe vera juice is an ideal toner for all skin types because of its astringent, antiseptic, healing and regenerative properties.

floral waters make soothing and healing skin tonics alone or as bases for
other ingredients. They are especially suited to very sensitive skin.

herbal infusions make great toners. Choose herbs suited to your skin
type (page 159).

herbal vinegars make very effective toners. The vinegar helps restore
the skin's pH and the herbs are cleansing, bracing and healing. Dilute
1 tablespoon (page 19) in 5 tablespoons of purified or floral water.

The following herbal infusions are best made fresh, unless otherwise stated.
Grapefruit seed extract will prolong their life span only a little, because
of their high water content. It is just as easy to make them fresh every
7–10 days, or to freeze batches in ice-cube trays and thaw as needed.

green tea & peppermint toner

FOR ALL SKIN TYPES

Green tea is high in anti-oxidants and protects the skin from free radical damage. It is helpful for all skin types, as is uplifting peppermint.

2½ tablespoons green tea infusion
2½ tablespoons peppermint infusion

+1

Mix the infusions and bottle.

healing floral toner

FOR ALL SKIN TYPES, ESPECIALLY SENSITIVE AND DEHYDRATED

This very fragrant, healing toner is one of my favourites. Use a floral water to suit your skin type (page 159). This toner will last for months in the fridge.

4½ tablespoons floral water
2 teaspoons aloe vera juice
10 drops grapefruit seed extract

Thoroughly combine the ingredients and store in the fridge.

elderflower water

FOR ALL SKIN TYPES, ESPECIALLY OILY SKIN WITH LARGE PORES OR PIGMENTATION

Elderflowers cleanse, tone and brighten the skin, and reduce pore size. Make a simple infusion of elderflowers (page 18), bottle and refrigerate.

honey & lavender toner

FOR ALL SKIN TYPES, ESPECIALLY OILY AND CONGESTED

This is a lovely healing and bracing toner.

¼ teaspoon honey
5 tablespoons witch hazel water
4 drops lavender essential oil

½ teaspoon apple cider vinegar

1 Dissolve the honey in the warm water.
2 Add the essential oil to the apple cider vinegar, then add to the honey water.
   Store in the fridge for up to six months. Shake well before each use.

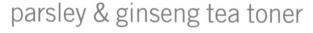

parsley & ginseng tea toner

FOR MATURE AND DEVITALISED SKIN

Parsley is high in vitamin C and ginseng promotes skin elasticity and epidermal cell production. This is sure to bring colour back to your cheeks!

2½ tablespoons parsley infusion
2½ tablespoons ginseng decoction

Mix the infusions well, bottle and refrigerate.

orange & fennel toner

Fennel seeds and fennel essential oil contain plant oestrogens, phytohormones that firm and rejuvenate the skin by stimulating the dermal cell metabolism. This lovely balancing, rejuvenating and fragrant toner is especially good for sluggish, untoned, lined skin, whether oily or dry.

½ teaspoon fennel seeds
5 tablespoons boiling water
2 teaspoons orange juice

43

1 Crush the fennel seeds using a mortar and pestle, cover with the boiling water
   and leave covered for 20 minutes
2 Strain the infusion, mix with the juice and bottle.

basil & lemongrass toner

FOR BLEMISHED SKIN

An infusion of basil leaves (page 18) makes a cleansing and toning freshener. Basil can help acne sufferers by killing bacteria on the skin. The scent of basil is also a known antidepressant, making it especially useful if you're feeling a little glum about your complexion. Lemongrass has impressive astringent properties and helps normalise the action of the oil glands.

sea of chamomile water

Chamomile has remarkable antiseptic and soothing qualities. The apple juice helps refine the skin.

4 tablespoons chamomile infusion
1 tablespoon apple juice

Mix the infusion with the juice and bottle.

jasmine & rose toner

FOR SENSITIVE. MATURE AND DEHYDRATED SKIN

This gentle and beautifully scented toner also makes a lovely perfumed body spray.

2½ tablespoons jasmine water
2½ tablespoons rosewater

Mix the floral waters well. Store in the fridge.

spirit soother toner

FOR ALL SKIN TYPES

A simple infusion of witch hazel makes an excellent cosmetic. It is high in tannic acid, a soothing and refreshing astringent, and can help reduce broken thread veins and large pores. It is
also antiseptic and can quickly reduce any kind of eye, face or body puffiness, which is why the
American Indians have used it for hundreds of years to bring down swelling from wounds.

black tea & lemon toner

Black tea is full of toning tannins and the skin saints – anti-oxidants. Lemon juice has acidic and astringent properties, helping remove deep-seated grease and grime, and leaving skin soft and clean. Lemon juice is also ideal for pimple-prone skin; it neutralises bacteria and boasts high levels of vitamin C, which helps heal skin. Use this toner only at night, as lemon can make the skin photosensitive.

5 tablespoons very weak black tea
2 teaspoons lemon juice

Combine the tea and lemon juice well, then bottle and refrigerate.

cucumber & gotu kola toner

FOR SENSITIVE SKIN

This lovely soothing, calming and brightening toner is especially beneficial for skin suffering from irritation, inflammation or fine surface capillaries.

½ cucumber, peeled
5 tablespoons gotu kola infusion

1 Juice the cucumber and strain.
2 Mix the juice with the infusion, bottle and refrigerate.

moisturisers

Moisturisers help prevent dehydration and dryness while creating a protective barrier against free radicals and moisture loss. Homemade moisturisers created with the rich and nourishing oils of fruits, nuts, seeds, vegetables, natural waxes, healing herbs and therapeutic essential oils are luxurious, anti-ageing treats that replenish, heal and revitalise the skin, leaving it calm, plump and succulent.

Moisturisers must contain both oil and water to keep the skin's surface layers soft and supple, and it is also important that they contain both emollients and humectants. Emollients – such as fat and oils – lock in moisture already present in the skin. Humectants attract water from the skin and the air and hold moisture in your cream and on your skin. A widely used humectant is glycerine, but honey is also effective. Ingredients best avoided are mineral oils and petrolatum (vaseline). Although they remove make-up, they end up sitting on the skin and causing pimples. They also offer no nutritional value, only robbing skin of its precious fat-soluble vitamins. A light cream replete with nutritious and readily absorbed ingredients is ideal. To add an SPF to your creams, substitute unrefined sesame oil, which has an SPF of 8, for the vegetable oils.

Moisturising is most important in the morning after cleansing and toning, to protect the skin from the vicissitudes of daily life. Resist burdening your skin with heavy creams at night, unless it is dry, as this is the one time the skin breathes and can excrete toxins. If your skin is very dehydrated or dry, apply a layer of aloe vera gel or a treatment oil under your moisturiser and sleep on it. Apply your moisturiser to a damp face and massage it in well. If there is any remaining moisturiser after 15 minutes, pat dry.

fresh milk lotions

Milk is a natural emulsion saturated with enzymes, vitamins, minerals and lipids. It comforts the skin naturally by increasing and retaining moisture levels, giving the complexion that smooth, creamy feel. Milk lotions are perfect for night wear, unless your skin is very dry. Apply with a cotton wool ball after cleansing and toning and sleep on it. In the morning your skin will feel soft and pulpy. Milk lotions should keep for up to 1 week.

mama's comforting milk lotion

FOR ALL SKIN TYPES

This comforting lotion will nurture tortured or neglected skin and is great when you're feeling a little sorry for yourself. Include dependable lavender in this preparation to encourage cell regeneration and sound sleep!

62 ml milk to suit your skin type (page 159)
½ teaspoon honey
½ teaspoon dried herbs (optional) or 1–2 drops essential oil to suit your skin type (page 159)

1 Pour the milk into a small saucepan, add the honey and herbs and bring to a simmer over low heat.
2 Simmer gently (do not boil) for 10–15 minutes.
3 Strain and refrigerate.

lemon & milk peel lotion with AHAs

This lotion is sure to refine, moisturise and brighten a dull, mottled, dry, flaky, oily or sallow complexion.

62 ml milk

2 teaspoons lemon juice

½ teaspoon vegetable glycerine or ½ teaspoon warmed honey

Combine the ingredients thoroughly and refrigerate.

oil lotions

jojoba moisturising oil

FOR ALL SKIN TYPES

The jojoba desert plant retains water during the long summer drought, and its waxy oil, pressed from the bean, does exactly that when applied to our skin. It provides a protective film over the skin and hair shaft, helping keep moisture in and free radicals out. Jojoba oil is very special and clever, and could almost be the extent of your beauty regimen – what more do you need when you have an oil that can cleanse, nourish, purify and protect the skin and hair? Queen of the oils, jojoba might seem expensive, but it's worth every penny. Another advantage of jojoba oil is that it is absorbed quickly by the skin and leaves no residue, so it can be used in all seasons. As jojoba tends not to turn rancid, this preparation will keep indefinitely.

2½ tablespoons jojoba oil
5–10 drops essential oil suited to your skin type (optional) (page 159)

1 Pour the oils into a bottle and shake well to mix.
2 Apply the oil to a damp face, leave for 15 minutes, then pat off any excess.

lime & cedarwood castile shaving oil

FOR ALL SKIN TYPES

My husband swears by this recipe.

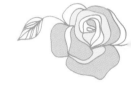

2½ tablespoons apricot kernel oil
2½ tablespoons Castile soap
6 drops lime essential oil
4 drops atlas cedarwood essential oil

1 Pour or drop all the ingredients into a bottle and shake well.
2 Always shake before use. Apply to warm, damp skin before shaving.

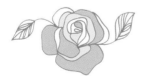

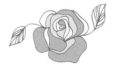

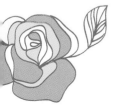

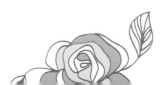

moisturisers

gel moisturiser

Gel moisturisers are hydrating, soothing and especially beneficial for oily or sensitive skin. I recommend them for sweltering summer days when the skin tends to become greasy.

never-an-oily-moment moisturising gel

FOR OILY SKIN

This soothing and hydrating gel doubles as a great after-sun treatment.

¼ teaspoon xanthan gum
5 tablespoons aloe vera juice
1 teaspoon vegetable glycerine
10 drops lavender essential oil

1 Using a small mixing wand, slowly mix the gum into the aloe juice until well dissolved and thickened.
2 Still blending, add the glycerine and essential oil. Store in the fridge for up to 1 month.

long-life emulsion moisturisers

These emulsions are similar to commercial moisturisers, except they contain only the purest of ingredients. They will keep for a long time, especially in the fridge.

calendula & rose moisturiser

FOR SENSITIVE SKIN WITH THREAD VEINS AND BROKEN CAPILLARIES

This is a lovely, medium-textured, healing and rejuvenating moisturiser for sensitive skin, with or without inflammation. It is also helpful for eczema and wrinkles.

oil phase
7 g plant-derived emulsifying wax
12 ml calendula infused oil
5 ml evening primrose oil
5 drops rosemary leaf extract

water phase
75 ml chamomile water
5 ml vegetable glycerine
12 drops grapefruit seed extract

third phase
20 drops rose essential oil (2.5 per cent dilution in jojoba oil)
5 drops German chamomile essential oil (optional)

Follow the instructions for making an emulsion on page 24.

the immortelle skin moisturiser

FOR DRY, SENSITIVE AND MATURE SKIN TYPES

One of the most impressive essential oils comes from the resilient yellow-petalled immortelle flower, also aptly known as everlasting, which grows wild in the sandy soils of the Mediterranean coast and possesses incredible powers of longevity – it never wilts. The oil extracted from this plant speeds up cellular growth and has formidable anti-inflammatory and anti-allergenic properties, making it wonderful for treating eczema and dermatitis.

oil phase

7 g plant-derived emulsifying wax

2 g shea or cocoa butter

15 ml calendula infused oil or sweet almond oil

5 ml rosehip oil

6 drops rosemary leaf extract

water phase

75 ml purified water or rosewater

5 ml vegetable glycerine

12 drops grapefruit seed extract

third phase

15 drops neroli essential oil (2.5 per cent dilution in jojoba oil)

5 drops immortelle essential oil

Follow the instructions for making an emulsion on page 24.

Other suggestions: rose and frankincense, combinations for mature skin (see page 157).

face

lavender & geranium moisturiser with rescue remedy

FOR NORMAL, OILY, DEHYDRATED, COMBINATION AND ACNEOUS SKIN

This is a lovely moisturiser for oily and dehydrated skin. Rescue Remedy is available at health food shops and makes an impressive healing addition if your skin is blemished, irritated or angry. Alternatively, you can use an essential oil combination suited to your skin type.

oil phase

6 g plant-derived emulsifying wax

10 ml jojoba oil

2 ml carrot infused or rosehip oil

4 drops rosemary leaf extract

water phase

85 ml purified water

5 ml vegetable glycerine

14 drops grapefruit seed extract

third phase

10 drops lavender essential oil

10 drops geranium essential oil

6 drops Bach Rescue Remedy (optional)

Follow the instructions for making an emulsion on page 24.

treatment oils

Facial oils can be used to help regenerate and boost the skin, while also treating a specific condition. A combination of cold-pressed vegetable oils and essential oils activates the skin to stimulate, heal, cleanse and tone.

Treatment oils are best used intermittently until the problem abates. Apply at night after cleansing and toning. If in the depths of winter your skin is feeling parched, you may want to apply a fine layer of moisturiser over the oil. If your skin is acneous, don't give up – you may have to apply nightly for at least 1–2 weeks before you see any results. An intensive treatment with toning oils at regular intervals is very beneficial for mature skin and can be used every night for a week, once a month.

For facial oils use a 1 per cent dilution (20 drops in 5 tablespoons of base oil) of essential oils. Use only 0.25 per cent dilution (5 drops in 5 tablespoons) if using long-term, to prevent the skin from becoming sensitised to a particular oil.

Pour the oils into a bottle and shake until well blended.

oil combinations

oily skin 5 teaspoons hazelnut oil, 5 teaspoons jojoba oil, 4 drops sandalwood essential oil, 3 mandarin, 3 palmarosa

dry skin 1 tablespoon sweet almond oil, 2 teaspoons avocado oil, 2 teaspoons olive oil, 2 teaspoons wheat germ oil, 4 drops sandalwood essential oil, 3 geranium, 3 rose

combination skin 5 teaspoons jojoba oil, 5 teaspoons sweet almond oil, 10 drops lavender essential oil, 6 geranium, 4 neroli

sensitive skin, eczema and dermatitis 5 teaspoons apricot kernel oil, 5 teaspoons jojoba oil, 3 drops chamomile essential oil, 3 atlas cedarwood, 2 lavender, 2 patchouli

dehydrated skin 1½ tablespoons apricot kernel oil, 1 tablespoon jojoba oil, 5 drops rose essential oil, 3 sandalwood, 2 palmarosa

mature skin 1 tablespoon jojoba oil, 2 teaspoons carrot root infused oil, 2 teaspoons evening primrose oil, 2 teaspoons rosehip oil, 6 drops rose essential oil, 3 frankincense, 2 patchouli

acneous skin 2½ tablespoons apricot kernel oil, 1 tablespoon jojoba oil, 2 teaspoons borage seed oil, 4 drops carrot seed essential oil, 2 chamomile, 2 lavender, 2 tea-tree

acne scars 1½ tablespoons jojoba oil, 2 teaspoons rosehip oil, 2 teaspoons wheat germ oil, 6 drops sandalwood essential oil, 4 lavender, 4 neroli

devitalised skin 2 tablespoons apricot kernel oil, 2 teaspoons wheat germ oil, 5 drops geranium essential oil, 3 rose, 2 cypress

broken capillaries 5 teaspoons apricot kernel oil, 5 teaspoons jojoba oil, 4 drops rose essential oil, 3 chamomile, 3 cypress

pigmentation 1½ tablespoons calendula infused oil, 1 tablespoon rosehip oil, 5 drops celery essential oil, 5 lavender, 5 lovage

treatment oils

exfoliants

Besides a bracing dip in seawater, exfoliating the face with a scrub, peel or cloth is the closest you'll get to achieving instant gleaming skin. In fact, there is little more satisfying in the realm of beauty rituals than seeing the skin promptly revitalised. Layers of dull, dead skin will be lifted gently, excess sebum and toxins removed and pores unblocked. This wonderful shedding process becomes increasingly important as we mature and our skin's ability to turn over cells decreases substantially.

While regular exfoliation is widely believed to be one of the keys to retaining and promoting a fresh, dewy, youthful complexion, you must be gentle. Even the slightest irritation or inflammation of the skin can provoke free radical activity, leading to premature ageing of the skin, so gently rub, don't scrub. To ensure your ingredients are ground down as finely as possible use a coffee grinder, but be sure to invest in separate grinders for your cosmetics and your coffee!

How often you exfoliate depends on the type of peel used, your work and your skin type. Once a week or a fortnight may suit sensitive skin, yet oilier skin may require gentle exfoliation every second day or even daily. Work in greasy kitchens or on dusty building sites will warrant regular, if not daily exfoliation. Winter life spent at home eating rich, fatty foods while huddled up to the heater will leave your skin feeling dry and unbalanced. Before spring, remove the accumulation of toxins and dead skin cells with more regular exfoliation.

Apply and massage exfoliants into a damp face with your fingers. Focus on clog-heavy spots around your nose, on your forehead and under your lower lip. Avoid the eye area and thread veins.

types of exfoliant

AHAs occur naturally in fruits such as citrus, apples and tomatoes. They also help dissolve dead skin cells, clearing the pores and revealing a brighter and more radiant complexion.

enzymatic peels contain enzymes that help dissolve dead skin cells, clearing the pores. Papaya and pineapple contain particularly effective enzymes for this purpose.

friction peels dry on the skin and are then gently rubbed off, removing the dead skin cells. These are suited to sensitive, fine and delicate complexions.

granular scrubs lift dead skin cells from the surface of the skin when rubbed. The granules can be made from ground nuts, seeds, grains and pulses. This type of exfoliant is especially beneficial for oilier, congested skin and blocked pores. They are also quite stimulating, benefiting dull, sluggish skin.

muslin (cheesecloth) wash cloths The gentle rubbing action of a muslin cloth exfoliates the skin while removing your cleanser.

washing pochettes Put some oatmeal and dried herbs in the middle of a piece of muslin (cheesecloth), tie up the corners, then moisten with lukewarm water and gently wash your face with it. This method works well for sensitive, fragile skin.

simple scrubs

basic scrub mix

FOR ALL SKIN TYPES

You may substitute any of the ingredients for other grains and seeds found in your cupboard, as long as they can be ground down very finely. Ground citrus zest, herbs and flowers to suit your skin type also make great additions to this base. For highly sensitive skin, omit the rice flour and double the oatmeal.

60 g very fine oatmeal
43 g rice flour
1 tablespoon clay suited to your skin type (page 11)

1 Combine the ingredients thoroughly and store in an airtight jar; the mix should last indefinitely if kept dry.
2 Put 2 teaspoons of the mixture in a bowl and add enough of a wet ingredient to complement your skin type (honey, yoghurt, milk, egg yolk, fruit, herbal infusions or floral waters – page 159) to form a gritty paste.
3 Spread the scrub onto a wet face and massage into the skin using gentle, upward circular motions. Remove with lots of tepid water and a muslin (cheesecloth) wash cloth. Repeat until all residue is removed. Pat dry.

Here are some exfoliants you can create with or without this basic scrub mix. If you haven't prepared the scrub mix, replace it with a finely ground grain or meal. Apply and remove the scrubs as for the basic scrub mix, unless otherwise stated.

papaya enzyme scrub

FOR ALL SKIN TYPES

Finely ground adzuki beans have the aroma of freshly cut grass. The Japanese use them to clarify the skin. They grind down to a beautiful and delicate consistency for exfoliation.

2 teaspoons mashed papaya
1 teaspoon ground adzuki beans

Combine the ingredients thoroughly.

the brightest hour strawberry scrub

FOR OILY AND COMBINATION SKIN (AVOID ON SENSITIVE SKIN)

This fine, fragrant, cleansing and balancing scrub will help clear oily, congested skin and brighten a tired, sallow complexion.

2 teaspoons basic scrub mix
1 teaspoon mashed strawberry
½ teaspoon natural yoghurt

Combine the ingredients to form a smooth paste.

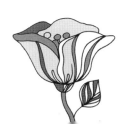

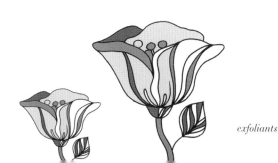

exfoliants

saving grace AHA scrub

FOR ALL SKIN TYPES

By combining a food boasting alpha-hydroxy acids with a grain of some sort in an exfoliant, you get the best of both worlds. The acids in the lemon and milk dissolve impurities, while the grains gently lift them.

1½ teaspoons basic scrub mix
½ teaspoon milk
½ teaspoon lemon juice

Combine the ingredients to form a smooth paste.

sushi scrub

FOR ALL SKIN TYPES, ESPECIALLY CONGESTED OR DEHYDRATED

This mineral-rich scrub with malic acid (an AHA found in apples) will help hydrate, smooth and soften the skin.

1½ teaspoons basic scrub mix
1 teaspoon apple juice
¼ teaspoon powdered kelp

Combine the ingredients to form a smooth paste.

sweet orange & almond scrub

FOR ALL SKIN TYPES

Bring the rose back into your complexion with this scrub. It is excellent for unplugging blocked pores and smoothing parched and flaky skin.

2 teaspoons almond meal
1 teaspoon honey
½ teaspoon orange juice

Combine the ingredients thoroughly.

banana silk scrub

FOR MATURE SKIN

The perfect antidote to skin chapped by harsh winter weather, this lovely nourishing and emollient scrub leaves the skin feeling soft and glowing. Avocado also works well in place of the banana.

1½ teaspoons basic scrub mix
1 teaspoon mashed banana
1 teaspoon cream
pinch ground cinnamon (optional)

Combine the ingredients to form a paste.

long-life exfoliants

These blends will slough off old skin, nourish, cleanse and brighten. They will last 3–6 months in the fridge.

sandalwood & mandarin face scrub

FOR SENSITIVE OR MATURE SKIN

Use this delightful, gentle scrub daily to slough off old skin, nourish, cleanse and brighten the complexion.

10 drops mandarin essential oil
5 drops sandalwood essential oil
70 g basic scrub mix

1 Add the essential oils to the basic scrub mix drop by drop, stirring constantly
   to avoid clumps.
2 Sift then store in an airtight jar.

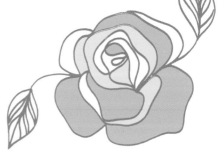

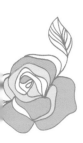

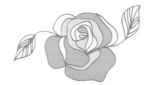

lemon & juniper clay scrub

FOR OILY, COMBINATION AND CONGESTED SKIN

Juniper is one of the most effective oils for treating congested and blemished skin.

10 drops lemon essential oil
10 drops juniper essential oil
70 g basic scrub mix

1 Add the essential oils to the basic scrub mix drop by drop, stirring constantly
   to avoid clumps.
2 Sift then store in an airtight jar.

herbal oats cleansing scrub

FOR OILY, COMBINATION AND CONGESTED SKIN

This delicious, thick and rich scrub will help clear the pores and prevent blackheads while nourishing the skin. This scrub will keep for up to 3 months in the fridge.

4 tablespoons fine oatmeal
2 tablespoons honey
3 teaspoons distilled witch hazel
1 teaspoon dried and ground peppermint
1 teaspoon dried and ground rosemary
1 teaspoon dried and ground sage
10 drops benzoin essential oil

Combine the ingredients thoroughly. Store in the fridge.

exfoliating balm

sticky butter cleansing balm

FOR ALL SKIN TYPES

I'd never considered making a cleansing/exfoliating balm until I had the pleasure of using UK facialist Eve Lom's cult Cleansing Cream, which is thick, creamy and absolutely delicious. It cleanses, exfoliates, moisturises and heals. It so inspired me that I decided to concoct my own version. With the help of Narelle Chenery, beauty guru and creator of Miessence, the first organic skincare company in Australia, I came up with this wonder balm. The key is to wipe the luscious, sticky balm away with warm water and a cotton cloth at least 3 times to remove thoroughly. Finish with a skin toner to eliminate excess grease. I also like to add dried and ground hops and dried and ground papaya to this recipe. Delicious!

20 g cocoa butter

12 g beeswax

4 tablespoons sweet almond oil

1 teaspoon honey

8 drops rosemary leaf extract

2 drops eucalyptus essential oil

2 drops peppermint essential oil

20 drops grapefruit essential oil

10 drops hops essential oil

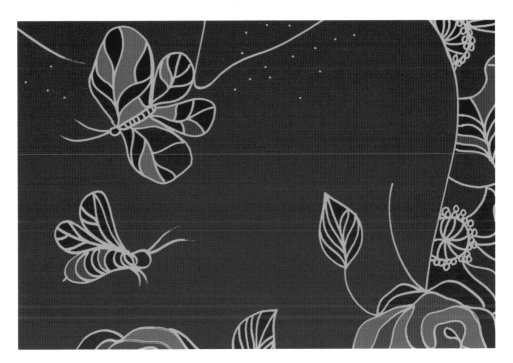

1 Slowly melt the cocoa butter, almond oil and wax in a bain-marie, stirring gently. Once melted, take off the heat.
2 When the mixture has cooled to body temperature, add the essential oils and rosemary leaf extract. Mix thoroughly.
3 Pour into jars.
4 Gently massage a small amount into the skin for a couple of minutes. Using a soft muslin cloth, or cotton flannel, and a sink full of tepid water, patting and pressing your face with the cloth, wipe away the balm. Wipe and rinse in this way three times. This balm will last up to six months.

masks

Creating your own wonderful, personalised face mask is akin to cooking a hearty and nourishing casserole without a recipe – rummaging through your cupboard to find anything that will complement the dish. Once you become familiar with the properties of ingredients and what they can do for your skin, you will have the freedom to whip up a mask on the spot.

My girlfriend came over recently with tired, greasy and devitalised skin. A couple of very angry spots protruded from her face and she was feeling a little downhearted. I took to the kitchen, apron on, beater and bowl in hand, and swung open the doors to my pantry and fridge to retrieve some remedies. I took a little apple juice mixed with honey, oats, clay, a splashing of wheat germ oil and a drop of lavender essential oil. I cleansed her face, applied a warm compress of water to soften the skin and then slathered on my mask mix from her forehead down to her collarbone. Once the mask was removed, her skin looked calmer and alive and, more importantly, she felt better. Masks not only revitalise the skin but the soul, inspiring time out and leaving you feeling relaxed and pampered.

It is believed that the first mask was invented by slave girls in Egypt who were washing their clothes at the Nile's edge. They realised that their feet became soft and pappy after immersion in the mud, and so decided to apply it to their face and hands. Since then, masks have evolved to include a plethora of ingredients that draw dirt, oil and impurities from the skin, soften blackheads, and cleanse, stimulate, soothe, soften, hydrate, balance, nourish, brighten, heal, revitalise and improve the colour, tone and texture of the skin. They can be made from a delicious mix of fresh fruit, veggies, herbs, oils, gels, clays, flours and essential oils.

How often you apply a mask depends on the condition of your skin and the type of mask. Normal skin may only need a purifying mask once a week or fortnight, whereas oilier skin will rely on more frequent applications. Mature or dry skin will benefit from a cleansing and nourishing mask at least once a week.

A mask is best applied to a well-cleansed face. For enhanced results, steam your face for 5 minutes before application and frame your face with a hair band to create the perfectly primed canvas. When pasting on face masks, skip any broken veins and the delicate skin around the eyes. Instead, coat your eyes with soothing slices of cucumber. Leave masks on for 10–15 minutes. If you have any excess mask, treat your décolletage too. Rinse off with lots of tepid water and a soft cotton cloth and follow with a toner and moisturiser.

types of mask

There are two basic types of mask:

drying masks which dry on the skin, and are predominantly extracting, purifying, stimulating and toning. Argiletz clays, fuller's earth, kaolin, egg and certain gels are common ingredients.

wet masks which infuse active ingredients into the skin, and hydrate, soothe, calm and heal. They usually stay wet on the skin and are often made from plants, fruit, vegetables, gels, dairy, herbs, egg yolks or honey.

impressive one-ingredient facials

avocado is a nourishing and smoothing treat for all skin, especially sensitive, dry and mature.

brewer's yeast stimulates and revives tired, dingy skin, and especially benefits oily complexions. Mix with warm water to form a paste and leave on the face for 10 minutes. Avoid on sensitive skin.

cabbage is a boon for treating inflamed, pimpled skin. Dip a couple of cabbage leaves into boiling water to soften them. Once cooled place them over your face for 10 minutes.

cornflour mixed with a little water makes a soothing mask, brilliant for calming irritated dry skin conditions like eczema.

honey spread in a fine layer over your face will help smooth and soften lines, treat skin eruptions, disinfect, cleanse, nourish and tone.

tahini a thick, buttery food made from pureed sesame seeds, softens and moisturises dry skin. Spread a fine layer over your face and leave for 10–15 minutes. Rinse off with a cotton cloth and lots of tepid water.

customise your mask

basic mask mix

FOR ALL SKIN TYPES

I use this basic mask for a lot of my facials. It is suitable for all skin types and contains healing, nourishing and purifying ingredients. You can add dried and ground herbs and flowers to suit your skin type.

60 g fine oatmeal
52 g clay to suit your skin type (page 11)
2 tablespoons almond meal

1 Combine the ingredients and store in a jar in a cool, dark cupboard.
2 Mix 1 tablespoon of the basic mix with several ingredients – eggs, yoghurt, milk, dried milk (especially for oily skin), vegetable oils, fruit, vegies, herbs, floral waters, herbal waters or essential oils (1–2 drops per mask) – to make a smooth paste. See page 159 for which ingredients best suit your skin type.
3 Don't let your mask become so tight that it starts to pull on the skin. Spray regularly with water to soften it. This mask may leave your skin a little red and warm but this should subside within a few minutes. Spray some floral water on your face to cool it down.

my favourite mask recipes

Here are some lovely mask combinations to pep up your complexion. If you don't like their runnier consistency you can set them with a little basic mask mix. If your skin is dry, it's a good idea to add some cold-pressed vegetable oil.

grandma's lemon tea mask

FOR UNTONED, DEVITALISED SKIN

An oldie but a goodie – this is a fine mask for oily skin that is feeling tired and dull and needs a little nurturing. It refines, tones, firms, smooths and brightens. If your skin is dry, replace the skimmed milk powder with full-fat milk powder.

1 teaspoon lemon juice
1 teaspoon strongly brewed tea, cooled
1½ tablespoons skimmed milk powder
1 teaspoon egg white, beaten until frothy

Add the lemon juice to the tea, then mix in the milk powder and egg white.

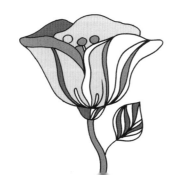

face

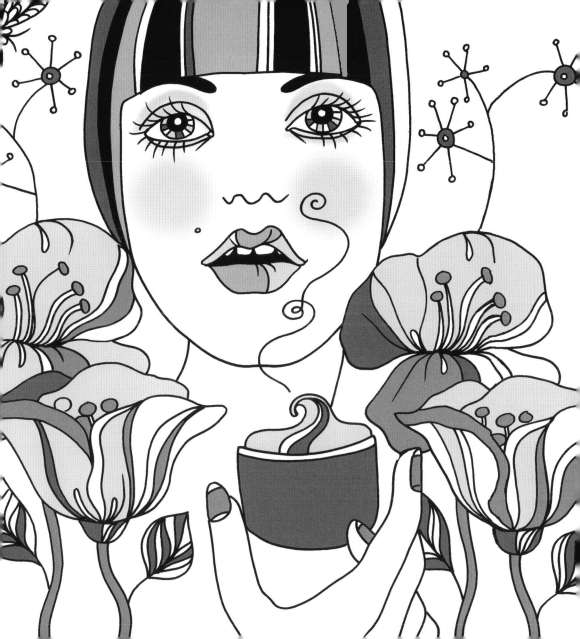

fresh herb mask

FOR ALL SKIN TYPES

This delightful mask will cleanse, tone and balance the skin. The live bacteria in the yoghurt will enhance your skin's health and balance.

1 teaspoon chopped fresh herbs to suit your skin type (page 159)
2 teaspoons natural yoghurt
2 teaspoons basic mask mix

Pound the herbs using a mortar and pestle and mix with the other ingredients.

AHA fruit gel mask

FOR DEHYDRATED, BLOTCHY OR CONGESTED SKIN

A fabulous exfoliating gel mask for unclogging the pores, this will also even up skin tone, improve hydration, and brighten and deep-cleanse the skin. Grape and lemon juice also work well.

2 tablespoons apple juice
1 tablespoon grapefruit juice
1 tablespoon strawberry juice
2 teaspoons citrus pectin

1 Combine the fruit juices.
2 Sprinkle the pectin over the juice mix then whisk to achieve the desired consistency.

olive & lime shine mask

FOR MATURE SKIN

This simple mask is full of anti-oxidants and AHAs that will soften and revive most complexions. If you wipe this mask off gently with a dry cloth, you'll be amazed at how much dirt it lifts! It works well as a 30-minute mask or left overnight and rinsed off in the morning.

2 teaspoons olive oil
½ teaspoon lime juice

Whisk the ingredients to combine until the mixture turns cloudy.

the amazing avocado & tomato mask

FOR ALL SKIN TYPES, EXCEPT SENSITIVE

This mask lightens and smoothes the complexion beautifully. Tomatoes are full of vitamins A, B and C, AHAs and the potent anti-oxidant lycopene, while avocado is rich in vitamins, good oils and lecithin.

2 teaspoons mashed avocado
2 teaspoons grated tomato pulp
2 teaspoons basic mask mix

Combine the ingredients thoroughly.

the korean bath house cucumber milk mask

At the Korean Baths in Sydney, they lavish a divine mix like this on my face while my body is being scrubbed. This is a delightfully hydrating, soothing and cooling mask.

2 teaspoons sweet almond oil
1½ teaspoons honey
1 tablespoon peeled and grated cucumber

Massage the oil into a clean face, spread the honey over the top, then pat the grated cucumber over the honey.

rose syrup mask

FOR OILY AND COMBINATION SKIN

This sweet-scented Ayurvedic mask is very popular among Indian women. It is balancing and toning for oily skin. Lemon juice is ideal for oily, blemish-prone skin because it is antibacterial and contains high levels of vitamin C, which help heal the skin.

1 tablespoon lemon juice
1 teaspoon rosewater
½ teaspoon honey

Combine the ingredients thoroughly.

lavender mud mask

FOR ALL SKIN TYPES, ESPECIALLY DEHYDRATED AND CONGESTED

Seaplants have been used for centuries for their healing properties by myriad cultures including the Chinese, Japanese and Polynesians. They boast the largest range of minerals of any organism and are used in skincare preparations for their cell-regenerative properties and their ability to attract and retain water. Aloe vera's cosmetic virtues have been extolled since biblical times. Together, these two ingredients make an exceptionally healing, calming, hydrating and regenerative mask that helps reduce the production of excess oil, resulting in a cleaner, clearer complexion with fewer breakouts. If your skin is very dry add a little avocado or olive oil. This mask is perfect for the advent of spring, when the body needs serious cleansing and detoxification.

1 tablespoon basic mask mix
3 teaspoons aloe vera juice
1 teaspoon kelp powder
1 drop lavender essential oil

Combine the ingredients thoroughly.

posh papaya mask

Papaya smooths out the skin splendidly without the need to lift a finger! It contains an enzyme called papain, which helps dissolve dead skin cells, thereby pepping up the most pallid of complexions. Macadamia nut oil contains palmatoleic acid found in human sebum, making it an excellent oil for mature and dry skin. Sandalwood is remarkably healing, hydrating and balancing, and has the headiest of scents. Spread this mask over your décolletage too. Don't throw the papaya seeds out, as they make a great remedial infusion for a facial steam.

76

1 tablespoon mashed papaya flesh
1 tablespoon basic mask mix
1 teaspoon macadamia nut oil
2 drops sandalwood essential oil

Thoroughly blend the ingredients.

smoothing honey mask

FOR DRY SKIN

When your skin needs a simple conditioning treatment, revive it with this lovely old-fashioned and well-known smoothing mix.

1 egg yolk, whipped
1 tablespoon powdered milk
½ teaspoon honey

Combine the ingredients well.

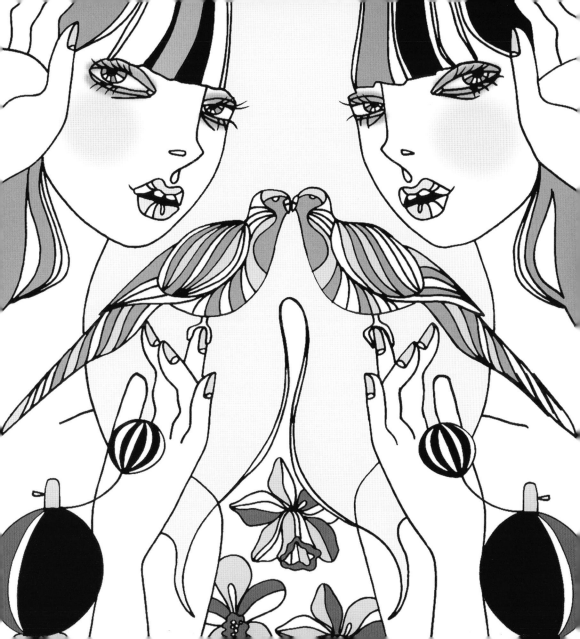

pear, sage & green tea cleansing mask

Pears have emollient properties and help moisturise, while green tea is anti-inflammatory and full of anti-oxidants. Sage is antibacterial, astringent, healing and also very cleansing, making it a wonderful anti-ageing ingredient.

1 tablespoon peeled and grated pear
1 tablespoon basic mask mix
1 teaspoon strong green tea infusion
1 teaspoon sage infusion

Combine the ingredients until the mixture is smooth.

78

manuka honey, carrot & bergamot mask

FOR ACNEOUS, IRRITATED AND ANGRY SKIN

This is an excellent remedial mask for troubled skin. Carrot juice is rich in skin-enhancing compounds, especially the anti-oxidant beta-carotene. Manuka honey boasts antibacterial properties 20 times stronger than those of tea-tree essential oil. The healing qualities and antidepressive scent of bergamot will help lift dull spirits and calm the complexion.

1 tablespoon basic mask mix
1 teaspoon carrot juice
1 teaspoon Manuka (or ordinary) honey
1–2 drops bergamot essential oil

Combine the ingredients until the mixture is smooth.

coriander mayonnaise mask

FOR DRY AND MATURE SKIN

My friend and natural health practitioner, Kevin Farrow, gave me this recipe. It is one of my favourites. I try to use it once a day for a week every month in winter, to keep my skin well fed.

1 egg yolk
½ avocado
½ bunch fresh coriander
1 tablespoon natural yoghurt
1 tablespoon orange juice
1 teaspoon rosehip oil

Combine the ingredients until the mixture is smooth.

chamomile, honey & orange blossom gel mask

FOR SENSITIVE SKIN

You can use other gelling agents, such as agar agar and xanthan gum, instead of pectin in this sweetly scented, gentle mask. It will cleanse and soothe sensitive skin.

2 teaspoons strong chamomile infusion
2 teaspoons orange blossom water
1 teaspoon honey
1 teaspoon pectin

1 Combine the infusion with the orange water, add the honey and mix thoroughly.
2 Sprinkle over the pectin and whisk until the mixture forms a gel.

aromatic ubtan cinnamon scrub mask

An Ubtan is a delicious mask made using grains, herbs and clay mixed with egg. It is pasted on the face and left to set. Then warm milk is spread over the top and the mix is gently rubbed off.This treatment is cleansing, stimulating and excellent for pepping up dull, sluggish skin. You can also use it to 'sand' the body, keeping it soft.

80

32 g basic mask mix
2 tablespoons sandalwood powder
2 teaspoons dried and ground rosehip
1 teaspoon ground cinnamon or nutmeg
1 teaspoon dried and ground orange zest

1 Combine the ingredients thoroughly and store in an airtight jar.
2 For normal and combination skin, mix 1 teaspoon with an egg yolk and egg white. For oily skin, mix 1 teaspoon with a whole egg white. For mature or dry skin, mix 1 teaspoon with an egg yolk.
3 Apply to the face and leave for 10 minutes.
4 Warm a little milk, massage into the mask, gently rub the mix off, then rinse.

miracle spice mask

FOR OILY SKIN

In India, where a tropical climate means oilier skin and a tendency to collect dust and grime, women herald fenugreek seeds as the miracle spice, with cleansing and rejuvenating properties.

1 tablespoon fenugreek seeds
2 tablespoons natural yoghurt

1 Soak the seeds in the yoghurt for an hour, then pummel with a pestle and mortar to make a smooth paste.
2 Gently rub the mixture onto the face and neck using circular movements. Leave on for 15 minutes, gently rub off, then rinse with water.

absolutely fabulous replenishing cream mask

FOR DRY AND MATURE SKIN

This mask is full of vitamins, fatty acids and anti-oxidants. Use once a week to revive the skin.

oil phase
9 g plant-derived emulsifying wax
2 g shea or cocoa butter
15 ml olive oil
5 ml rosehip oil
6 drops rosemary leaf extract

water phase
65 ml rosewater
5 ml vegetable glycerine
12 drops grapefruit seed extract

third phase
10 drops lavender essential oil
10 drops frankincense essential oil

Follow the instructions for making an emulsion on page 24.

vitamin c peel pack

Freckles and dark patches on our skin are usually caused by the sun's rays. Any inflammation of the skin can also make it more susceptible to pigmentation, so it's important to keep the skin calm, well nourished and protected. Regular exfoliation is effective, as it helps remove dead cells, allowing a fresher, brighter and more evenly toned skin to emerge. Citrus fruits, strawberries, tomatoes, milk and yoghurt boast skin-brightening AHAs. Papaya and pineapple also boast excellent skin-refining enzymes. Vitamin C used topically is reputed to reduce pigmentation.

82

⅛ teaspoon soluble vitamin C powder (ascorbic acid, preferably with bioflavonoids)
2 teaspoons papaya juice
2 teaspoons pineapple juice
1½ tablespoons basic mask mix
1 drop lemon essential oil (optional)

1 Dissolve the vitamin C in the combined papaya and pineapple juices.
2 Blend the vitamin mixture with the mask mix to form a smooth paste.
3 Add the essential oil and mix well.
4 Apply to the face and decolletage, leave for 15 minutes, warm a little milk, massage into the mask, then rub the mix off. Rinse well.

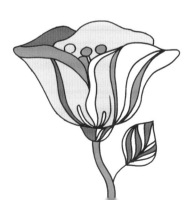

lady muck's pre-party facial

To pep up the complexion just before going out, you want a treatment that will calm, nourish, tone and brighten it, not bring out impurities.

1 egg white
1 teaspoon strong chamomile infusion, cooled

83

1 Whisk the egg white until a little foamy then add the chamomile infusion.
2 Apply lightly with a brush.
3 Leave on for 15 minutes, then rinse off gently with lots of tepid water and a cotton cloth.

long-lasting clay masks

These masks are wonderfully therapeutic and will keep for up to 1 year in the fridge.

deep-cleansing & balancing clay mask

FOR OILY CONGESTED SKIN

4 drops orange essential oil
3 drops palmarosa essential oil
3 drops sandalwood essential oil
26 g green clay

1 Add the oils to the clay drop by drop and mix thoroughly.
2 Sift the mix to remove clumps.
3 Combine 1½ teaspoons of the mix with enough water, herbal infusion, honey
   (preferably Manuka) or floral water to make a smooth paste.

calming rose & chamomile mask

FOR SENSITIVE SKIN, WITH OR WITHOUT BROKEN CAPILLARIES

This strengthening mask will help calm, tone, decongest and heal the skin while reducing redness and blotchiness.

6 drops rose essential oil (2.5 per cent dilution in jojoba oil)
4 drops chamomile essential oil
26 g pink clay

1 Add the oils to the clay drop by drop and mix thoroughly.
2 Sift to remove any clumps.
3 Combine 1½ teaspoons of the mix with enough rosewater, herbal infusion and/or honey to form a paste. For dry skin, use a cold-pressed vegetable oil or egg yolk.

spot treatments

one-ingredient treatments

FOR ACNEOUS SKIN

To treat blemishes, rub them with nasturtium or calendula (marigold) petals, or coat them with a layer of honey and rinse with warm water after an hour then rub lightly with highly antiseptic garlic cloves.

bust-my-spot treatment

Out damn'd spot! This is a very effective zapping treatment for pimples.

1 tablespoon myrrh tincture
5 drops lavender essential oil
5 drops lemon essential oil
5 drops tea-tree essential oil

Mix the ingredients thoroughly and apply a small amount to individual blemishes
(not the whole face!).

85

turmeric paste

FOR DAMAGED SKIN

Turmeric is excellent for wound-healing, for bruises and as a decongestant. Mixed with water
to form a paste, it also dries out pimples. Leave on for a couple of hours or overnight. Exfoliate
the skin gently to remove the stain.

tomato juice & green clay paste

FOR ACNEOUS SKIN

Mix about 1 teaspoon of green clay with about ½ teaspoon of tomato juice to form a paste.
Tomatoes are high in vitamins A, B and C and AHAs. Together with the extractive properties
of green clay, tomato juice makes a formidable mask for spots or acneous patches.

lips

Lips are hard little workers, contorted many times each day as we express ourselves and, more importantly, exchange warm feelings through a blessed kiss. Without an effective lipid barrier, our lips lose moisture regularly, and their lack of melanin (our body's own protection against sun damage) and sebaceous glands makes them prone to drying out, chapping and developing infections such as cold sores. To sport soft, plump lips, it is vital to wear a natural, protective and vitamin-enriched lip balm daily. To keep moisture trapped, it's important that your lip preparations contain a humectant like glycerine or honey, or a protective emollient like jojoba.

Most commercial lip preparations are made from petrochemicals, such as petroleum jelly and mineral oils – not to mention myriad other nasty chemicals. The following lip balms and exquisite lip tint are made from natural, health-promoting ingredients like vegetable oils, waxes, extracts, butters and essential oils. You will also find that you don't need to reapply zillions of times throughout the day. Pucker up and enjoy!

lip treatments

exfoliation To keep your lips in good shape, exfoliate regularly and gently with a soft children's toothbrush or damp flannel.

honey To help smooth the lips, layer resinous honey over them and leave for 15 minutes or longer.

vitamin E A few drops rubbed into the lips and left overnight make a wonderful nourishing and healing treatment.

cold sore healing preparation

5 drops geranium essential oil
5 drops lavender essential oil
5 drops tea-tree essential oil
1 tablespoon myrrh tincture

1 Add the essential oils to the tincture, bottle and shake well to mix.
2 Apply the preparation sparingly to the cold sore throughout the day.

lip balms

making a lip balm

The natural properties of beeswax soften and protect lips, making it the ideal ingredient for a moisturising lip balm. Your essential oils, in a maximum dilution of 20 drops for every 100 g of balm, should be non-toxic and should not photosensitise the skin. Here is a basic balm-making method to use with the recipes that follow.

1 Melt the beeswax and/or cocoa butter and/or shea butter in a bain-marie.
2 Add the vegetable oil and/or honey, keeping the mixture over heat.
3 Using a small mixing wand, beat well to blend the ingredients.
4 Remove from heat and, once the mixture begins to cool, stir in any essential oils.
5 Pour into small jars, lipstick moulds or pretty tin pillboxes.
6 For a lovely shine, use a lip brush to apply.

basic healing lip balm

10 ml vitamin E oil (tocopherol)
50 ml jojoba oil
10 g beeswax

Mix the vitamin E into the jojoba oil then follow the instructions for making a lip balm above.

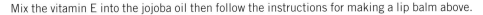

mandarin & anise lip gloss

Anise has a delicious aroma, reminiscent of licorice. It has reputed aphrodisiac powers and helps allay frazzled nerves. Mandarin will also help calm the mind.

12 g beeswax
8 g cocoa butter
50 ml calendula infused oil
½ teaspoon honey
9 drops mandarin essential oil
6 drops anise essential oil

Follow the instructions for making a lip balm opposite.

lime & sandalwood healing lip balm

Shea butter is a wonderful emollient that offers natural sun protection.

15 g beeswax
5 g shea butter
50 ml jojoba oil
5 ml calendula infused oil
8 drops lime essential oil
7 drops sandalwood essential oil

Follow the instructions for making a lip balm opposite.

lip tint

beetroot & orange lip & cheek tint

Put the healing lip balm on top of this for a shiny pink pout.

2 teaspoons beetroot powder or crystals
3 teaspoons vodka
¼ teaspoon vegetable glycerine
3 drops sweet orange essential oil

1 Dissolve the beetroot powder in the vodka.
2 Add the glycerine and oil, mixing well.
3 Apply with a brush. Store in a bottle for up to 3 months in the fridge.

eyes

The delicate skin that cradles the eyes is stretched, twisted and puckered up countless times a day as we laugh, weep, squint at bright lights, wince at dusty city air, blink to keep our eyes moist and, as the evening approaches, struggle to keep our peepers open. Because this skin boasts fewer oil glands than the rest of the face, it is far more prone to lines and wrinkles.

Regular application of eye creams, gels and oils will help prevent, reduce and smooth out cracks and crevices and keep the skin plump and moist. Rich and heavy creams will only drag the skin down in that area, exacerbating already existing lines and creating new ones, so opt for feather-light creams and apply them gently around the orbital bone, using the kind middle finger. Try not to be too critical of those fine character lines – the eyes are the windows to our soul and a few laughter lines surrounding them can be an endearing and welcoming feature.

Avoid commercial eye gels or toners that contain alcohol – they may temporarily tighten the area but are harsh and cause all sorts of skin irritation. Certain herbs will help other common problems, like dark circles and bags.

eyebright

As its name indicates, eyebright has long been used to add a special shine to eyes. Mix 20 drops of tincture of eyebright into a glass of chilled distilled water and apply morning and night to closed eyes using cotton wool balls.

puffiness & dark circles

finger treatment

Puffiness around the eye can be reduced by gently patting the bone around the eye with a finger (middle is best).

the magic spoon treatment

One of my favourite tricks is to put stainless steel spoons in the freezer for 10 minutes and then place them over my eyes for a few minutes. This is a fabulous way of reducing puffiness before going out or after a late night.

potato treatment

To lighten dark circles and tighten skin, wrap a grated raw potato in muslin (cheesecloth) and apply to eyelids for 15–20 minutes. Gently wash off any residue then apply a light eye cream or jojoba oil.

fresh food remedies

Here are some effective ways to combat puffy panda eyes using fresh ingredients.

buttermilk tones under the eyes, helping restore the acid mantle.

cucumber tones up the skin around the eyes and cools and soothes inflamed eyes. Peel a piece of cucumber and squeeze the juice right into your eye, or use a slice of peeled cucumber as an eye pad.

teas Place wet chilled tea bags or cotton balls soaked in tea over closed irritated, gritty and puffy eyes. Black, calendula, chamomile, fennel, green, parsley, red clover and rosehip teas all work well.

fresh fig on closed eyes will reduce puffiness.

fresh cold milk Soak cotton wool balls in milk and place over closed eyes for 10 minutes.

witch hazel Chill and apply to closed eyes using cotton wool balls.

more eye treatments

eye pillow

The weight of an eye pillow will help reduce inflammation and puffiness of the eyelids. Join two 10 × 20 cm pieces of pure silk on three sides to make an envelope. Pour 1 cup of uncooked rice into the opening and add some dried lavender flowers to make it fragrant and calming. Sew up the gap.

eyewashes

To ensure that your eyebath is perfectly clean, dip it in boiling water before and after use. Eyewashes should always be made fresh as needed. Any of these infusions may be used as an eyewash for sore, tired, irritated and 'gritty' eyes: borage, calendula, chamomile, elderflower, fennel seed and parsley.

To use, fill an eyebath with a weak warm herbal infusion or decoction strained and filtered through coffee filter paper. Use cool if there is any swelling. Hold the eyebath over the eye, tilt back your head and blink rapidly several times. Roll your eyes around and pat dry with a clean cloth.

eye soothers

regenerative eye oil

FOR ALL SKIN TYPES

Rosehip oil is very popular in regenerative skincare. It is extracted from the fruit of a rose bush that grows wild in the southern Andes and is extremely beneficial in tissue regeneration for burns, facial wrinkles and scars, probably due to its high concentration of fatty acids. Rosehip oil makes an excellent night oil for mature skin, and also those with oily skin, because of its high content of both fatty acids and trans-retinoic acid. I often add a couple of drops of immortelle essential oil to this mix, as it seems to help diminish dark circles. This oil will keep for up to 1 year.

2 tablespoons jojoba oil
2 teaspoons rosehip oil
5 drops immortelle essential oil (optional)

1 Pour or drop the oils into a bottle and shake well to combine.
2 Moisten the skin around and under the eye. Pat on a few drops of the oil using the middle finger of your chosen hand. Keep patting gently until most of the oil is absorbed. Leave for 20 minutes and then blot off any surplus oil.

soulful eye cream

FOR ALL SKIN TYPES 95

This is a light moisturising cream for around the eyes. Rose and carrot seed oil both improve skin tone and elasticity and help prevent wrinkles.

oil phase
7 g plant-derived emulsifying wax
10 ml apricot kernel oil
5 ml rosehip oil
4 drops rosemary leaf extract

water phase
80 ml rosewater
5 ml vegetable glycerine
14 drops grapefruit seed extract

third phase
5 drops carrot seed essential oil
10 drops rose essential oil (2.5 per cent dilution in jojoba oil)

Follow the instructions for making an emulsion on page 24.

eye mask

soothing cucumber milk mask

This is a lovely, gentle, soothing and slightly toning eye mask.

2 teaspoons peeled and grated cucumber

1 tablespoon powdered milk

1 teaspoon honey

1 Combine the ingredients to form a paste.
2 Apply over and around closed eyes. Leave for about 10 minutes then rinse with cool water and follow with the regenerative eye oil (page 94).

body

all over

Ruddy décolletages and coarse, parched body skin are often caused by lack of moisture, poor diet and not enough protection from the sun's rays. Mediterranean cultures have always recognised the importance of sustaining the body with nourishing foods that can counteract the damaging effects of a hot climate. In Greece, pomegranate, one of the most potent anti-ageing fruits, is still revered for its protective qualities. It contains three times the anti-oxidants of green tea. When eaten or applied topically, this bejewelled fruit helps ravage free radicals, preventing them from wreaking havoc in the body and on the skin. A well-known recipe made by Greek women is a delicious body butter of macerated pomegranate, beeswax and olive oil. They apply this rich mixture all over their bodies each day to ensure healthy, gleaming skin.

If your temple is looking a little broken or weathered, some love, attention and fresh food therapy will help rebuild its beautiful and unique structure. Remember, a wholesome diet and lots of exercise and relaxation are your temple's supporting pillars. Shun harsh chemical cleansers that strip the skin, and lavish organic foods, essential oils and nutritious ingredients on your precious self to feed, nurture and revitalise your body.

body cleansers

make-me-over body cleanser

FOR ALL SKIN TYPES

This gentle foaming cleanser will leave your body fragrant, soft and squeaky clean. It will last up to 6 months in a cool place, away from direct sunlight. For extra healing and cleansing properties, add 2 teaspoons of a clay that suits your skin type (see page 11).

4 tablespoons liquid Castile soap
2 teaspoons sweet almond oil
20 drops essential oil (optional)

Pour or drop the ingredients into a bottle and shake well to combine. Shake well before each use.

Depending on your mood, try one of these essential oil combinations: *relaxing* – 8 drops bergamot, 8 lavender, 6 chamomile; *refreshing* – 8 drops orange, 6 grapefruit, 6 lime; and *antiseptic* – 8 drops geranium, 8 lavender, 6 tea-tree.

body buffing

Buffing the body with a natural-bristle brush or natural homemade body scrub is probably the quickest way to achieve healthy, lustrous skin. As the skin on the body is much tougher than on the face, you can scrub firmly, using bigger, sharper granules, like sugar and salt. Blemishes on the body, like those on the face, reflect a deficiency in the diet or toxicity. So while following these delicious recipes will be of assistance, it's also important to reassess your lifestyle.

all over

dry skin body brushing

FOR ALL SKIN TYPES

This very old and revered technique not only whisks away built-up dead skin cells, but kick-starts the lymphatic system, helping to eliminate a generous portion of the body's waste. It helps diminish the appearance of cellulite, and tone flabby areas of the body. I always feel like I've been for a good half-hour walk after brushing for a few minutes.

Stand bare in a comfortable space and stretch your whole body from the tips of your toes to the top of your head to awaken the senses. Starting at the feet, make long sweeping strokes over the front and backs of the legs. Brush over the bottom and up to the mid-back. Brush your hands, arms, across the shoulders, up the neck, down the chest (skipping the nipples!) and down to the tummy. Using circular motions, brush the abdomen in a clockwise direction. Remember: always work towards the heart and then stroke downward, pushing toxins toward the colon. Follow with a warm shower, finished with 10 seconds of cold water. Avoid brushing too vigorously or you may scratch the skin. If the skin on your body is very sensitive, invest in a soft-bristled brush.

body scrubs

Body scrubs feel wonderful and relieve itchy, flaking skin. Salt and sugar are both perfect bases to which to add vegetable oils, infused oils, herbs and essential oils, as they do not create a big sodden mess like grains. Apply all scrubs to a damp body, massage into the skin, then rinse well.

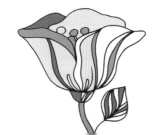

body

fresh ginger scrub

The Japanese have used this scrub for centuries. Mix 2 teaspoons of grated ginger with 2 tablespoons of sea salt and rub into cellulite to decongest fatty deposits and improve circulation.

salt & pepper scrub with coffee, cinnamon & orange

FOR SPONGY AREAS ON THE THIGHS AND BOTTOM

Coffee stimulates and dispels congestion, and grapefruit essential oil stimulates the lymphatic system, promoting the removal of wastes and toxins.

120 g sea salt
26 g white clay
1 teaspoon ground coffee
1 teaspoon ground cinnamon
1 teaspoon dried and ground peppermint leaves
15 drops grapefruit essential oil
15 drops orange essential oil

1   Combine the dry ingredients thoroughly.
2   Add the essential oils drop by drop, mixing well to avoid clumps.
3   Store in an airtight jar in the fridge for up to 1 year.
4   Combine 2 tablespoons of the mix with enough water, milk or oil to form
    a smooth paste, then massage into the body.

all over

celtic salt body scrub

FOR ALL SKIN TYPES, EXCEPT VERY SENSITIVE

This simple salt scrub polishes to perfection. Poppy seeds and honey make fabulous additions to this scrub. Warning: oily preparations can make the shower recess very slippery!

240 g celtic or finely granulated sea salt
20–40 drops essential oil of your choice (optional; see the oil combinations on page 113 for ideas)
125 ml sweet almond or other cold-pressed vegetable oil

1 Pour the salt into an airtight preserving jar.
2 Add the essential oils to the base oil drop by drop and blend.
3 Pour the oil mixture into the salt. Seal the jar and shake well. This mixture will keep for up to 6 months.

pink tangerine, rosewood & lavender scrub

FOR SENSITIVE SKIN

This also makes a balancing body mask; leave on for 20 minutes then rinse thoroughly.

120 g fine oatmeal
2 tablespoons pink clay
2 teaspoons dried and finely ground chamomile flowers
10 drops lavender essential oil
10 drops tangerine essential oil
10 drops rosewood essential oil

1 Drop the oils into the clay.

2 Sift out any wet clumps.

3 Add the oatmeal and the chamomile flowers. Store in an airtight container.

4 Combine 3 tablespoons of the mix with enough water or milk to form a paste.

green clay scrub with salt, rice, bergamot, lavender & ylang-ylang

FOR OILY OR BLEMISHED SKIN

Without the salt, this makes a clarifying body mask for oily skin.

86 g rice flour

3 tablespoons sea salt

2 tablespoons green clay

10 drops bergamot essential oil

10 drops lavender essential oil

6 drops ylang-ylang essential oil

1 Drop the oils into the clay.

2 Sift out any wet clumps.

3 Add the rice flour and the sea salt. Store in an airtight container.

4 Combine 3 tablespoons of the mix with enough water or milk to form a paste.

body masks

When planning to dress your body in a mask, make sure you have enough time, space, privacy, towels and running water before you start – the simplest tasks can be difficult to negotiate when you're smothered in a thick layer of goo.

olive oil anti-oxidant mask

FOR ALL SKIN TYPES, EXCEPT VERY OILY

Olive oil is full of anti-oxidants and makes a wonderfully nourishing and strengthening skin treatment. Slather a thoroughly cleansed body with olive oil, then pop on some old cotton clothes for 1 hour. Take the clothes off and your body will be soft and pulpy. You don't need to wash the oil off; by the time it has been absorbed by both your clothes and skin there shouldn't be any left.

sundari body mask with avocado & rose geranium

Sundari means 'beautiful woman' in Sanskrit. Make fresh as needed.

2 tablespoons green clay
1½ tablespoons papaya
1 teaspoon avocado oil
5 drops rose geranium essential oil

1 Combine the ingredients to form a paste.
2 Spread over a clean, damp body, leave for 10–15 minutes, then rinse.

brown rice miso & honey body paste

Genmai or brown rice miso mixed with honey makes a rich and delicious body paste. Miso is full of skin-smoothing amino acids. Extend this to your face for a nourishing treat.

2 tablespoons honey
1 tablespoon brown rice miso

1 Combine the ingredients to form a smooth paste.
2 Spread over a clean, damp body, leave for 10–15 minutes, then rinse well.

the very kind banana & marshmallow body scrub or mask

FOR SENSITIVE SKIN

This lovely scrub or mask will cleanse and hydrate the skin, improving tone and texture. It is also wonderful for relieving itchy, flaky skin. Marshmallow is anti-inflammatory and very soothing. Make fresh as needed.

3 tablespoons basic scrub or mask mix
2½ tablespoons marshmallow decoction (or chamomile infusion)
2 tablespoons mashed banana
2 tablespoons natural yoghurt

1 Combine the ingredients thoroughly.
2 For a scrub, massage gently over the body then rinse off. For a mask, apply to a clean, damp body, leave for 20 minutes then rinse.

all over

papaya skin-rub mask

FOR ALL SKIN TYPES

To dissolve dead skin cells and soften the skin, rub the insides of a papaya skin all over a clean, damp body. Leave for 20 minutes then rinse off.

bridal body mask

FOR ALL SKIN TYPES

I was given this wonderful mask recipe by my friend Yasmin Sadikot, the pioneer of Ayurvedic treatments in Australia. It is traditionally used by Indian brides, who prepare it 10 days before the wedding and apply it every day until the ceremony for soft, clear, fragrant skin.

4 tablespoons finely ground wheat germ
2 tablespoons ground almond meal
1 tablespoon dried and ground orange peel
1 tablespoon dried and ground lemon peel
1 tablespoon ground thyme
½ tablespoon ground turmeric
pinch salt
2 drops rose or jasmine essential oil

1 Combine the dry ingredients thoroughly.
2 Add the essential oil drop by drop and mix well.
3 Store in an airtight jar.
4 Combine 3-4 tablespoons of the mix with enough sweet almond oil to form a smooth paste, spread over a clean, damp body and leave for 20 minutes. Firmly rub off the dried mask and rinse well.

deluxe cream mask

FOR MATURE SKIN

Slather a layer of cream all over your body and leave for 15 minutes to soak in. To enhance its softening properties, add a splash of lemon juice.

body moisturisers

Keep the body nourished and supple with these wonderful moisturising preparations.

frankincense, bergamot rind & lime body lotion

FOR ALL SKIN TYPES

This uplifting, soothing, hydrating and non-greasy lotion is easily absorbed by thirsty skin.

oil phase
9 g plant-derived emulsifying wax
2 g cocoa butter
20 ml sweet almond oil
6 drops rosemary leaf extract

water phase
170 ml purified water, floral water or aloe vera juice
8 ml vegetable glycerine
34 drops grapefruit seed extract

all over

third phase

18 drops bergamot essential oil

18 drops lime essential oil

12 drops frankincense essential oil

Follow the instructions for making an emulsion on page 24.

very french floral body balm

FOR MATURE, DRY SKIN

Ylang-ylang, patchouli and rose make a divinely scented suit. Ylang-ylang has a balancing effect on skin, making it ideal for all skin types. Ylang-ylang's jasmine-like, heavy and intense fragrance is a renowned aphrodisiac. Patchouli and rose are also renowned as inspiring good loving!

oil phase

16 g plant-derived emulsifying wax

10 g cocoa butter

40 ml sweet almond oil

5 ml evening primrose oil

12 drops rosemary leaf extract

water phase

120 ml rosewater

8 ml vegetable glycerine

25 drops grapefruit seed extract

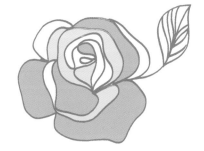

third phase

15 drops patchouli essential oil

15 drops palmarosa essential oil

10 drops neroli essential oil (2.5 per cent dilution in jojoba oil)

10 drops ylang-ylang essential oil

Follow the instructions for making an emulsion on page 24.

body powder

Body powders absorb perspiration and moisture from the skin, making them ideal for balmier weather, when clothes tend to rub against sweaty skin and cause chafing and irritation. Body powders can also be dusted over the body after a shower or bath to help speed up drying time and to lightly scent the body. Powders of arrowroot, cornflour (cornstarch), orris root flour, potato flour, rice flour and white clay can be used alone or in combination.

basic dusting powder

FOR ALL SKIN TYPES

To make a deodorising powder for under the arms, add ¼ cup of bicarbonate of soda (baking soda) to this combination. Orris root comes from the Florentine iris and boasts a beautiful delicate scent, reminiscent of violets.

52 g white clay powder

72 g fine cornflour (cornstarch) or orris root powder

20 drops essential oil of your choice

all over

1 Combine the dry ingredients in a completely dry blender.
2 Add the essential oil drop by drop and blend until mixed thoroughly.
3 Sift to remove any lumps. Decant the powder into a salt or parmesan shaker for easy dusting onto the body, or use a powder puff to apply.

Here are some deliciously fragrant essential oil combinations for your powder: *sensual and spicy* – 10 drops orange, 8 sandalwood, 2 cinnamon; *soft lavender* – 8 drops bergamot, 6 lavender, 6 natural vanilla essence; *exotic floral* – 8 drops rose, 7 jasmine, 5 ylang-ylang; *uplifting* – 10 drops lavender, 6 geranium, 4 nutmeg; *deodorising* – 9 drops lemon, 6 patchouli, 4 myrrh; *citrus* – 12 drops grapefruit, 6 bergamot, 4 orange; and *spring flowers* – 6 drops palmarosa, 4 rosewood, 2 geranium.

deodorants

The pheremones released in our sweat may influence both who we attract and who we are attracted to, and yet we quash this natural body chemistry with the use of deodorants. Your body odour is far less offensive if your body is healthy. Natural deodorants do not prevent perspiration, which is important, because sweating out unwanted toxins is necessary for healthy body function. Instead, they mask the odour and may inhibit the growth of bacteria.

Sage was popularly used by the Chinese to control body odour and lovage was a favourite deodorant among the ancient herbalists. Other effective deodorising herbs are basil, calendula, eucalyptus, lavender, lemongrass, mint, rosemary, sage, spearmint, tea-tree, thyme, yarrow, or any other appealing pungent herb. For a deodorant, make a 50 per cent dilution in water of a herbal vinegar made with a combination of these herbs. All green leafy vegetables are high in chlorophyll and can be rubbed into the armpits to reduce perspiration odour. If your odour is pungent, try rubbing some watercress or parsley under your arms before spritzing with the following spray. Bicarbonate of soda (baking soda) is also very effective.

arabian nights deodorant spray

FOR ALL SKIN TYPES

Patchouli essential oil has been used by the Arabs for years to hide body odour, and cypress is renowned for quashing wetness. This spray has a sweet, heady and sensual aroma.

3 tablespoons distilled witch hazel
2 tablespoons vodka
2 teaspoons glycerine
15 drops bergamot essential oil
15 drops citrus seed extract
10 drops lime essential oil
10 drops patchouli essential oil
5 drops cypress essential oil

Combine the ingredients and store in a spray bottle in the fridge for up to 1 year.

body oils

A body massage is one of life's most pleasurable experiences – we all need to be touched and nurtured by other human beings. A massage has many health benefits: it stimulates the circulatory and lymphatic systems, increasing the elimination of toxins and improving muscle and skin tone; and it arouses and soothes the nervous system, resulting in a feeling of well-being and relaxation.

Vegetable oils are nourishing and can be used alone or with essential oils. They are the perfect vehicle for carrying essential oils deep into the skin and throughout the whole body. This penetration takes around 20 minutes.

To prevent deterioration of your oil, add 10 per cent vitamin E oil. Recommended massage base oils are sweet almond, apricot kernel, sunflower, safflower, soybean, olive and jojoba.

herbal infused oils

Herbal infused oils make wonderfully therapeutic massage oils. Choose herbs to suit your skin type (page 159) and follow the instructions for making an infused oil on page 20.

the very orange blossom body spray

This is a delightfully fragrant and uplifting orange-scented body spray. Neroli oil is extracted from the white blossoms of the bitter orange tree, petitgrain from the leaves of the bitter orange tree and sweet orange from the peel of the orange.

10 drops neroli essential oil
10 drops petitgrain essential oil
10 drops sweet orange essential oil
2 tablespoons vodka
3 tablespoons orange blossom water

1　Stir the essential oils into the vodka, then mix with the orange blossom water.
2　Pour into a spray bottle. Shake well before each use.

aromatherapy massage oils

For a typical aromatherapy massage mix 15–25 drops of essential oil with 3 tablespoons of carrier oil. Here are some suggestions: *energising* – 10 drops grapefruit, 8 bergamot, 4 peppermint; *detoxifying and stimulating* (good for cellulite) – 10 drops grapefruit, 8 lemon, 6 juniper; *toning* – 6 drops cypress, 6 lemon, 6 patchouli, 6 rose; *relaxing* – 10 drops sandalwood, 8 neroli, 8 rose; *for lovers* – 10 drops orange, 6 patchouli, 4 cinnamon, 4 ylang-ylang; and *for pregnancy/stretch marks* – 5 drops lavender, 5 mandarin.

cocoa massage bars with mandarin, lime & nutmeg

Use this as a massage bar, or cut off a sliver and pop it in your bath. Massage it into cuticles, heels and elbows.

70 g cocoa butter

5 g beeswax

1 tablespoon coconut oil

15 drops lime essential oil

15 drops mandarin essential oil

4 drops nutmeg essential oil

1 Melt the cocoa butter, beeswax and coconut oil in a bain-marie and mix well.

2 Remove from the heat for a few minutes then add the essential oils.

3 Pour into moulds then refrigerate to harden. Store in the fridge.

jasmine infused body gloss

The warm, heady perfume of jasmine is synonymous with love and sex; it is mentioned in the Kamasutra as a fragrance that penetrates the five senses. It increases the beta waves in the brain, making you more aware of everything around you. At the end of winter and beginning of spring, when jasmine is starting to bloom, I put jasmine petals in a bottle of apricot kernel oil and infuse them for 10 days (page 20). Sometimes I throw dried mandarin peel into the mix to give a little citrus flavour to this floral oil. It makes a lovely skin gloss for balmy evenings out. To enhance the fragrance, add a few drops of jasmine and mandarin essential oils. Ylang-ylang, neroli, sweet orange, patchouli and sandalwood also work well.

caribbean spice body oil

This lovely woody, aromatic body oil for both sexes can be used on the body or as a bath oil.

2 whole cloves
1 cinnamon stick
1 large bay leaf, crushed
1 vanilla pod, split and cut into pieces
125 ml jojoba oil
30 drops sweet orange essential oil (optional)
10 drops patchouli essential oil

1 Infuse the herbs and spices in the jojoba oil for 2 weeks (see page 20).
2 Strain through coffee filter paper.
3 Add the patchouli oil and the sweet orange oil if using.
4 Leave to mellow for 2 weeks before use.

insect repellant

don't bug me

I have an aversion to most commercial insect repellents, which usually contain a whole host of dubious synthetic chemicals. Certain essential oils are extremely good at repelling little critters; I like to add them to a balmy base that will roll onto the skin easily. If you prefer a spray, use the Arabian Nights deodorant spray base (page 111) to carry the essential oils below. Citronella and lemon are also impressive insect repellents. Damp green tea leaves rubbed on insect bites will help relieve itching. Fresh basil leaves or fresh slices of onion will also relieve stinging.

15 g beeswax
10 g cocoa butter
3½ tablespoons sweet almond oil
20 drops geranium essential oil
20 drops lavender essential oil
15 drops lemongrass essential oil

1 Melt the beeswax and cocoa butter in a bain-marie, mixing well to combine.
2 Remove from heat for a few minutes, then add the essential oils.
3 Pour into a mould then allow to solidify at room temperature. Store in the fridge.

all over

neck

The neck is one of the first places to show signs of ageing. Engage in regular neck excercises to firm up those defiant muscles, and apply a nourishing and firming mask weekly. Extend your facial toners, exfoliants and moisturisers to your neck, using light, upward, feathery strokes.

herbal neck toners

Stimulate the extra-dry, wrinkled areas of the neck with herbal infusions that have astringent properties. Suitable herbs are horsetail, lime flower, nettle, peppermint, sage or thyme.

replenishing neck and breast oil

FOR ALL SKIN TYPES

This lovely light oil will help keep the neck toned and moisturised.

2 tablespoons apricot kernel oil
1 tablespoon jojoba oil
1 tablespoon rosehip oil
8 drops neroli essential oil (2.5 per cent dilution in jojoba oil)
6 drops lavender essential oil
4 drops frankincense essential oil

1 Pour or drop the oils into a bottle and shake to combine.
2 Massage into the neck using upward, circular motions.

hands

We anoint our faces and necks with the finest concoctions to help keep them soft and succulent, but neglect to pamper our diligent and tactile old paws, which are constantly on display to the world. My grandmother once rightly said that a woman's hands give her age away quicker than her face. The skin on the hands lacks oil glands, and so is very prone to dryness and premature ageing. Add years of washing in solvents, sun exposure and general wear and tear, and they are likely to shrivel up and develop conditions like dermatitis. To protect them and keep them soft and pappy, slip on cotton gloves under your rubber set when washing up to prevent perspiration and irritation. When gardening, opt for reinforced fabric gloves. Avoid using harsh soaps, and apply a homemade hand cream after washing to replace lost moisture.

hand cleansers

rough silk hand cleanser

FOR ALL SKIN TYPES

Keep a small jar of coarse oatmeal near the sink. Spoon 1 teaspoon into the palm of your hand, mix with water and rub your hands together thoroughly to cleanse. Add 5 drops of lavender oil to the jar for a fragrant and antiseptic cleanse.

grapefruit soap cleanser

FOR ALL SKIN TYPES

This is a lovely refreshing and antiseptic foaming cleanser.

2½ tablespoons Castile soap
1 teaspoon olive oil
10 drops grapefruit essential oil

Pour or drop the ingredients into a bottle and shake well to combine.

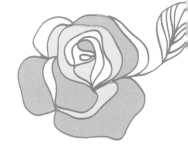

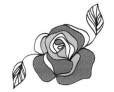

hand scrubs

sugar & lime hand scrub

FOR ALL SKIN TYPES

This lovely weekly treat for dry, flaky, dull and mottled hands will smooth and brighten. It smells sweetly of freshly peeled lime zest.

4 tablespoons granulated raw sugar
2 tablespoons sweet almond oil
10 drops distilled lime essential oil

1 Combine the ingredients thoroughly and store in an airtight jar.
2 Massage 1 teaspoon of the mixture into dampened hands, then rinse.

quickie lemon & olive scrub

FOR ALL SKIN TYPES

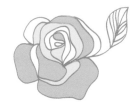

1 tablespoon granulated raw sugar
2 teaspoons lemon juice
2 teaspoons olive oil

1 Combine the ingredients thoroughly.
2 Rub onto damp hands then rinse.

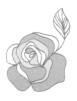

hand moisturisers & masks

patchouli in wintertime hand oil

FOR ALL SKIN TYPES

Dry midwinter hands will revel in this heavenly scented oil. Smother them in it, leave for 15 minutes and pat off the excess. Or slip your oily hands into cotton gloves and sleep on it.

1½ tablespoons olive oil
1 tablespoon avocado oil
5 drops patchouli essential oil
5 drops rose essential oil
2 drops benzoin essential oil

Combine the oils thoroughly and store in a bottle.

softening clay & honey hand mask

FOR ALL SKIN TYPES

1½ tablespoons white clay
1 tablespoon natural yoghurt
2 teaspoons honey

1 Combine the ingredients thoroughly.
2 Spread over the hands, leave for 10–20 minutes, then rinse off.

non-greasy lavender & rosemary moisturiser

FOR ALL SKIN TYPES

This is the hand cream to have with you at all times.

oil phase
8 g plant-derived emulsifying wax
2 g cocoa butter
2 teaspoons sweet almond oil
2 drops rosemary leaf extract

water phase
4 tablespoons purified water, aloe vera juice or lavender water
1 teaspoon vegetable glycerine
16 drops grapefruit seed extract

third phase
10 drops lavender essential oil
10 drops rosemary essential oil

Follow the instructions for making an emulsion on page 24.

121

honey hand-steaming mask

FOR ALL SKIN TYPES

When your hands are looking like worn animal paws, slather them in honey then steam them for 5–10 minutes over a bowl of hot water containing emollient and healing herbs, like licorice root, chamomile, elderflower, calendula and marshmallow root. Rinse with oatmeal in water and then apply a moisturiser. Slip on a pair of cotton gloves and sleep on it.

hands

liver spot hand mask

FOR MATURE SKIN WITH UNEVEN PIGMENTATION

Liver spots appear with age and as a result of accumulated exposure to the sun. They respond well to regular exfoliation and foods rich in AHAs and vitamin C. Bicarbonate of soda has a bleaching effect. Shield the hands from the sun with an SPF sunscreen to prevent further pigmentation. See also the pigmentation treatment oil on page 55.

2 teaspoons lemon juice

2 teaspoons bicarbonate of soda (baking soda)

2 teaspoons powdered buttermilk

1 Combine the ingredients thoroughly.
2 Spread over the hands, leave for 20–30 minutes, then rinse off. Apply twice a week until you notice a difference. Follow with a protective hand cream.

nails & cuticles

The condition of the nails and cuticles depends on a healthy diet rich in vitamins and minerals. Harsh chemicals, chlorine from swimming pools, overuse of nail enamel and nasty acetone-based polish removers, as well as other aggressive external factors, can wreak havoc on your nails, causing brittleness, splitting and ragged cuticles, hangnails and infection. I find that the contents of a vitamin E capsule or a touch of wheat germ oil massaged into the nails and cuticles daily is a wonderfully simple preventative treatment.

nail soaks

To strengthen nails, soak them in a herbal infusion of horsetail for 5 minutes daily. The stems of the horsetail plant are rich in silica: vital for healthy nails, bones and hair. Apple cider vinegar is also effective; soak your fingertips in a shallow bowl for 5 minutes. Buttermilk is a wonderful cleanser, nourisher and softener; soak your nails in it, then push back the cuticles with a wooden cuticle stick covered in cotton wool.

123

nail-strengthening oil

FOR WEAK OR BRITTLE NAILS

Most commercial nail strengtheners work by drying out the nails' vital oils, making them brittle. Soaking your nails in a good vegetable oil is a much healthier option. This mixture can be massaged into nails morning and night to keep them flexible and strong, and prevent brittleness, hangnails and ragged cuticles. It will also stimulate circulation, therefore encouraging better growth.

2 tablespoons sweet almond oil
2 teaspoons vitamin E oil
15 drops lemon essential oil
10 drops frankincense essential oil

1 Combine the oils thoroughly.
2 Massage into the skin at the base of the nail and over the nail itself.

nail-fix oil

FOR NASTY NAIL INFECTIONS

2 tablespoons wheat germ oil
10 drops palmarosa or tea-tree essential oil
10 drops spike lavender essential oil

1 Thoroughly combine the oils and store in a small bottle.

2 Rub a few drops into the infected area 3 times a day until the infection clears.

pineapple & yolk nail softener & cuticle exfoliant

This wonderful nail and cuticle softener and conditioner will help dissolve any dead skin and nourish at the same time. If you don't have any pineapple juice, use another acidic juice like apple, tomato, grape, lemon or orange juice.

2 tablespoons pineapple juice
1 tablespoon egg yolk

1 Combine the ingredients.
2 Massage into the cuticle area, leave on for a couple of minutes, then rinse off.

dirt cleanser

To get rid of ingrained dirt under the fingernails, dig them into lemon halves then scrub vigorously with apple cider vinegar.

nail polishes

Toluene and formaldehyde, used widely in commercial cosmetic polishes, can cause throat irritation, rashes, headache, nausea and asthma. But if you are partial to a little polish, there are a few good natural alternatives.

Try buffing your nails with beeswax, cocoa butter or a tiny amount of vegetable oil and a soft cloth. Naturally buffed and nicely shaped nails look luxuriously pampered. Buffing is good for your nails, as it stimulates circulation in the nail bed, helping the nails get stronger. Be sure to buff them in an up-and-down motion, as this stimulates blood flow and creates a glorious sheen.

seashell polish

Mix some henna powder with water to make a paste, apply a 1 millimetre layer to clean dry nails, then leave to dry in the sun or dry with a hair dryer – the warmth will intensify the colour. Rinse off and dry the nail. Buff to a high polish and your nails will resemble pretty pink sea shells. Run a white pencil under the nail tips to accent them and create the effect of a French polish. Henna is a marvellous conditioner for the hair and nails; it will prevent both from splitting and give them a glorious shine.

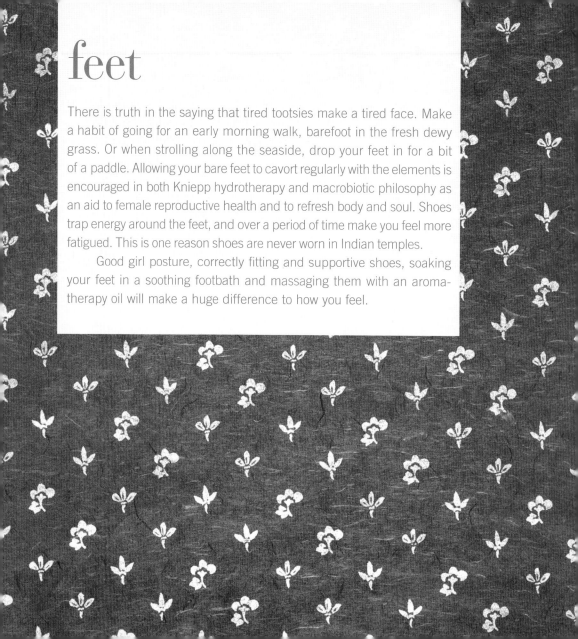

feet

There is truth in the saying that tired tootsies make a tired face. Make a habit of going for an early morning walk, barefoot in the fresh dewy grass. Or when strolling along the seaside, drop your feet in for a bit of a paddle. Allowing your bare feet to cavort regularly with the elements is encouraged in both Kniepp hydrotherapy and macrobiotic philosophy as an aid to female reproductive health and to refresh body and soul. Shoes trap energy around the feet, and over a period of time make you feel more fatigued. This is one reason shoes are never worn in Indian temples.

Good girl posture, correctly fitting and supportive shoes, soaking your feet in a soothing footbath and massaging them with an aroma-therapy oil will make a huge difference to how you feel.

reflexology

The ancient healing art of reflexology is based on the belief that every organ of the body is connected to reflex points in the foot, hand or ear. By massaging the feet for 10 minutes each day you are helping to release any blockages in the body and to bring it into balance.

Start out by kneading the soles firmly. The big toe is said to represent the head; gently pull each big toe and carefully rotate it – this will help relieve a stiff neck and tense shoulders. Use both hands to wring out your foot like a damp cloth and tap it to stimulate circulation. Squeeze the area above the heel, around the ankle, which is said to represent the reproductive organs, and press down firmly on any sore points.

aromatherapy foot oil

20 drops essential oils
5 tablespoons sweet almond oil

Add the essential oils to the almond oil and mix thoroughly. Store in an airtight bottle.

Some suggested essential oil combinations are: *warming* – 14 drops grapefruit, 3 ginger, 3 clove; *cooling and energising* – 10 drops mandarin, 6 lemongrass, 4 peppermint; *relaxing* – 8 drops lavender, 8 orange, 4 ylang-ylang; and *for fungal infections* – 20 drops palmarosa, 20 thyme, 10 myrrh.

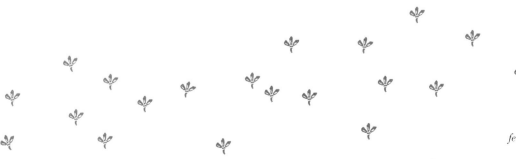

feet

reviving rosemary & lavender foot & leg massage oil

An infused oil of rosemary and lavender (page 20) makes an excellent massage oil for the feet.

foot scrubs & masks

Any ground grain or flour works well on the hard parts of the foot when mixed with a cold-pressed vegetable oil. Salt and sugar scrubs are wonderfully invigorating and slough off tough bits superbly. On hot summer days at the beach, use the rough granules of sand and softening sea water to exfoliate your feet. The simplest way to remove dead skin from the feet and prevent the skin from cracking is to scrub them regularly with a pumice stone. Follow with a refreshing foot scrub.

overnight heel-softening treatment

To remove a build-up of hard, dead skin, soak feet for 15 minutes in a warm to hot footbath containing 2 tablespoons of bicarbonate of soda (baking soda). Pat feet dry, then rub over a mixture of ¼ cup of olive oil and 2 tablespoons of apple cider vinegar. Pop on your socks and sleep on it.

lemon-half heel scrub

FOR ALL SKIN TYPES

To soften and whiten rough elbows and heels, fill empty lemon halves with sugar, place your elbows or heels in them and rub firmly.

salt, kelp, lemon & clay foot & body scrub

This is a delicious antibacterial, softening and detoxifying foot scrub. You can vary the essential oils as follows: *skin-strengthening and circulation-improving* – geranium; *antiseptic, antifungal and uplifting* – lemon. The kelp will help soften and smooth the skin.

215 g medium-textured sea salt
1 tablespoon green clay
1 teaspoon powdered kelp (optional)
20 drops lemon or lemon myrtle essential oil

1 Combine the ingredients together well and store in an airtight container.
2 Combine 2 tablespoons of the mix to form a gritty paste. Massage into the feet using circular motions, paying particular attention to areas with built-up hard skin.

warming coconut & spice foot paste

Massage this smoothing, softening, uplifting and sensual paste all over the feet and body. Essentail oils of jasmine, rose, patchouli and ylang-ylang can be added for an exquisite aroma.

1½ tablespoons coconut milk
2 tablespoons oatmeal
2 teaspoons sweet almond oil
1 teaspoon mixed spice

1 Combine the ingredients to form a smooth paste.
2 Massage over the feet, leave for up to 20 minutes, then rinse off.

footbaths

A good old-fashioned foot soak makes a wonderful alternative to a body bath. Soaking your feet for 10–15 minutes relaxes and revives and has myriad therapeutic properties. It helps reduce swelling, prevents varicose veins, treats cellulite and quells any fire in the mind. Herbs, oils and salts make wonderful therapeutic additions to footbaths.

cold Stand in cold water up to your calves for 2 minutes in the morning. This will invigorate your body and mind in preparation for the day.

lemon A footbath of 125 ml lemon juice (or vinegar) in a basin of water will revive the feet, relieve itchiness and treat athlete's foot.

pebbles For a tactile, sensuous soak, rub your feet slowly and firmly over a dozen or so small stones placed at the bottom of your favourite footbath.

honey & ginger footbath

Ginger promotes circulation and is very warming for winter. Add 2 teaspoons of ground ginger and 2 tablespoons of honey to a bowl of hot water. This is also an excellent remedy for a thick, unrelenting head cold, or for warding off a chill.

herbal deluxe deodorising footbath

The warmth and sweat generated by the feet provide the perfect environment for bacteria to grow, often leading to smelly feet. Thankfully, they can be treated with good foot hygiene and the frequent use of deodorising footbaths and foot powders. This wonderfully soothing and invigorating bath will freshen up even the most tainted of tootsies. Other effective deodorising herbs are basil, bay leaves, eucalyptus, lemon balm, lemongrass, lovage, marjoram, parsley, spearmint and thyme. Black tea laced with lemon juice also works wonders, and lemon and orange peel make wonderful healing and fragrant additions.

2 tablespoons dried lemon zest
3 teaspoons dried lavender
2 teaspoons dried peppermint leaves
2 teaspoons dried rosemary leaves
2 teaspoons dried sage leaves

1 Add the ingredients to a half-filled hot footbath and let the herbs infuse for 20 minutes.
2 Fill the bath with hot water and soak your feet for 10 minutes.

deodorising footbath with essential oils

This combination will help diminish perspiration and leave the feet smelling like they've just frolicked through an evergreen forest.

8 drops rosemary essential oil
6 drops cypress essential oil
6 drops pine essential oil
2 tablespoons vodka
1 tablespoon cold-pressed vegetable oil

1 Drop the essential oils into the vodka and stir well.
2 Pour the mixture into a basin of hot water.
3 Add the vegetable oil and swish around.
4 Adjust the temperature with hot or cold water and soak your feet.

soothing bath salts

Lavender is a natural pain reliever with relaxing and analgesic properties, while geranium and orange reduce swelling and help the body unwind. The clay will impart enhanced healing properties.

215 g Epsom salts
1 teaspoon green clay (optional)
20 drops orange essential oil
10 drops geranium essential oil
10 drops lavender essential oil

1 Combine the dry ingredients.
2 Add the essential oils drop by drop, stirring until well mixed.
3 Transfer to an airtight jar and leave for a week before using.
4 Add 2 tablespoons to a basin of warm water.

back-to-your-roots footbath

When you're feeling a little lost in superficial matters or your mind is off with the pixies, draw a footbath and lace it with these grounding essential oils: 8 drops lavender, 6 patchouli, 6 sandalwood. Mix well.

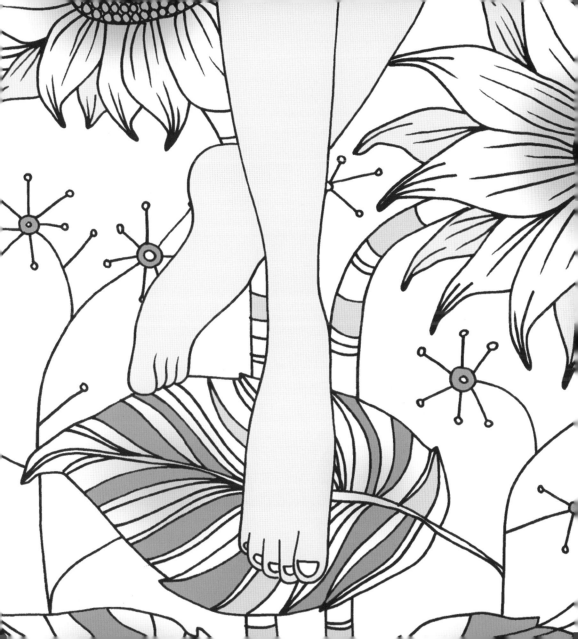

foot powders

Homemade foot powders are a superb alternative to talcum powder. Cornflour (cornstarch), potato flour, arrowroot flour, rice flour, orris root flour and white clay are all ideal, used individually or together. They absorb moisture and perspiration and can be brushed alone over the feet to ease blisters and help remedy fungal infections like athlete's foot (especially bicarbonate of soda). Dried herbs and essential oils make fabulous additions. The following powders will last up to 1 year in the fridge.

absolutely fabulous foot powder

36 g cornflour (cornstarch) or orris root powder
68 g bicarbonate of soda (baking soda)
52 g white Argiletz clay (or kaolin)
2 tablespoons herbs and flowers, dried and ground (optional)
20 drops essential oils

1 Combine the flour and bicarbonate of soda with the clay and herbs (if using).
2 Add the essential oils drop by drop, stirring constantly.
3 Sift then store in a tightly lidded container with holes punched in the top, or in a salt or parmesan shaker. Shake well before each use.

Here are some essential oil suggestions: *for fungal infections* – 8 drops lavender, 8 tea-tree, 4 lemon; *refreshing and deodorising* – 8 drops cypress, 6 bergamot, 6 grapefruit; *earthing and healing* – 8 drops orange, 6 geranium, 6 patchouli; or *invigorating* – 10 drops lavender, 6 rosemary, 4 spearmint.

moisturisers

peppermint & mandarin foot cream

Keep your feet smooth with this cooling, soothing and easily absorbed moisturising cream.
It will last for up to 1 year in the fridge.

oil phase
7 g plant-derived emulsifying wax
3 g cocoa butter
15 ml sweet almond oil
5 drops rosemary leaf extract

water phase
75 ml purified water
5 ml vegetable glycerine
12 drops grapefruit seed extract

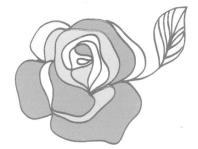

third phase
25 drops mandarin essential oil
5 drops peppermint essential oil

Follow the instructions for making an emulsion on page 24.

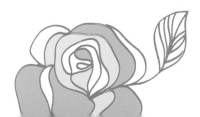

rich lavender, lemongrass & shea butter hand & foot treatment balm

This is a rich balm for dry, cracked and damaged hands and feet. Myrrh's healing properties have long been revered. Calendula is also exceptionally effective on rough, callused skin.

oil phase

9 g plant-derived emulsifying wax

2 g shea butter

5 g cocoa butter

20 ml calendula infused oil

6 drops rosemary leaf extract

water phase

60 ml rosewater

5 ml glycerine

10 drops grapefruit seed extract

third phase

15 drops lavender essential oil

5 drops myrrh essential oil

5 drops lemongrass essential oil

Follow the instructions for making an emulsion on page 24.

hair

Your crowning glory or an unruly tangle? The condition of your hair is a good barometer of your state of health and wellbeing (although with the amount of dying, straightening, curling, blow-drying and harsh products we inflict on our tresses, it would be hard to tell!). Your nails, skin, teeth and hair are always last in line when your system distributes nutrients, so you must eat a well-balanced diet if you want lovely hair. Lack of sleep, stress and sad spirits will also manifest themselves in dull, lifeless hair and sometimes in hair loss.

The first step towards shiny, lustrous hair is to banish harsh shampoos. Like skin, hair is naturally acidic, and regular washing with alkaline shampoos will upset the acid balance and damage your tresses. Many people I know have ceased using such shampoos and have found that their dandruff and hair loss have eased.

Your hair will be full of residues from the chemical formulations you have been using, so it will take a little while for natural treatments to remove this build-up, and for your hair to feel soft and look shiny.

handy hair tips

head & scalp massage

Massaging the hair and scalp stimulates the body's systems, including the glands, nerves and circulation, promoting hair growth and reducing dandruff.

oil treatments

Jojoba oil lubricates, improves shine and lustre, restores damaged hair, strengthens the hair shaft and treats scalp imbalances. Other vegetable oils are also beneficial, including apricot kernel, castor, coconut, olive and sweet almond oil. Massage into the hair and scalp and cover with a plastic shower cap or cling film and a warm, damp towel. Leave for 30 minutes to allow the oil to penetrate the hair shaft. Rinse then shampoo.

diving for pearls hair oil

To protect your hair from salt or chlorine, rinse your hair in fresh water before plunging into a pool or the ocean. Or apply a little of this exquisitely scented oil to protect hair from the sun or sea. Pearl divers wear ylang-ylang oil in their hair for this reason.

2 tablespoons coconut oil
2 tablespoons jojoba oil
10 drops ylang-ylang essential oil

Pour or drop the oils into a bottle and shake well to combine.

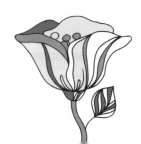

hair clean-up

To eliminate shampoo build-up rinse your hair with ½ cup of bicarbonate of soda (baking soda) in 1 cup of warm water. Rinse well. Soda water also works well as a hair rinse.

dandruff

mr snowman's dandruff treatment

Dandruff can be caused by a number of things, such as an inadequate diet, insufficient brushing, shampoo build-up, aggressive hair products and bad scalp circulation. Avoid medicated shampoos; they may relieve dandruff in a day or so, but it will often come back worse than before. Use once a week.

2½ tablespoons jojoba oil
8 drops lavender essential oil
6 drops rosemary essential oil
6 drops tea-tree essential oil

1 Combine the oils thoroughly.
2 Massage into clean, damp hair and scalp and cover with a plastic shower cap or cling film and a warm, damp towel. Leave for 1–2 hours.
3 Rinse thoroughly, shampoo, then rinse in apple cider vinegar (1 tablespoon in 1 cup warm water). Condition if required.

hair loss

Hair loss may happen gradually or in clumps. Male pattern baldness is pretty hard to fight, but can be relieved with many stimulating and nourishing ingredients.

hair replenishing oil

FOR THINNING HAIR

This mixture may slow hair loss. Use once a week.

2½ tablespoons jojoba oil

10 drops atlas cedarwood or clary sage essential oil

10 drops rosemary essential oil

1   Pour or drop the oils into a bottle and shake well to combine.
2   Massage into damp, clean hair, and leave on for at least 30 minutes or overnight.
3   Rinse thoroughly with warm water; shampoo and condition as normal.

hair treatment oils

Combine 2½ tablespoons of jojoba oil or another vegetable oil with these essential oil combinations and massage into the hair to help treat your hair condition. Use at least once a week and leave for at least 30 minutes or overnight. Also use them in your base shampoos: *normal hair* – 15 drops geranium, 15 lavender; *oily* – 20 drops bergamot, 10 patchouli; *dry* – 15 drops sandalwood, 15 ylang-ylang; and *fragile* – 15 drops carrot seed, 15 lavender.

dry fragrant hair oil

This sensual blend of oils will keep your hair lustrous and healthy.

20 drops jojoba oil
10 drops sandalwood essential oil
5 drops bergamot essential oil
5 drops clary sage essential oil
5 drops jasmine essential oil
5 drops rose essential oil

1   Combine the oils thoroughly.
2   Place 3 drops on the fingertips and/or on your hairbrush and run through your hair.

shampoos

Many commercial shampoos contain sodium lauryl sulfate, a skin irritant, so ensure that your shampoo is sulfate-free. Most homemade shampoos do not lather like bought shampoos, but will keep your hair as clean and in excellent condition. Shampoo your hair only when it really needs it, and use lukewarm water for shampooing and cold water for the final rinse.

quickie shampoo

FOR ALL HAIR TYPES

Buy a mild, pH-balanced, sulfate-free shampoo base at a health food shop and add 20 drops of essential oil for every 5 tablespoons of shampoo.

fragrant yolk & castile conditioning shampoo

Eggs have been used to cleanse and condition hair for generations because of their cleansing and moisturising properties. This is a fabulous simple, fragrant conditioning shampoo for all hair types. I use this recipe often to revive and add lustre to my hair. It also tames fly-aways.

½ teaspoon liquid Castile shampoo base
1 egg yolk
2 drops essential oil to suit your hair type (page 163)

Combine the ingredients thoroughly.

dry shampoo

FOR ALL HAIR TYPES

Flours absorb impurities from the hair, get rid of that greasy look and are great when you can't shampoo your hair. White clay and orris root powder also work very well.

10 drops essential oils of your choice
36 g cornflour (cornstarch)

1 Add the essential oils to the cornflour drop by drop, mixing thoroughly to avoid clumps.
2 Sift.
3 Massage small quantities into your hair, close to your scalp. Use a brush to distribute the mixture and to begin to remove it, then tip your head upside down and continue brushing to remove the rest.

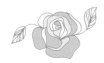

clay shampoo with orange & ylang-ylang

FOR OILY HAIR

This cleansing and balancing shampoo will also help whisk dead skin away from the scalp.

5 tablespoons shampoo base
2 teaspoons green clay
10 drops orange essential oil
10 drops ylang-ylang essential oil

Combine the ingredients thoroughly.

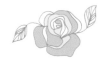

conditioners

Conditioners are especially useful if your hair has been over-permed, over-coloured or other-wise abused. When your body is healthy and balanced and you are using gentle, natural shampoos, you may find that you don't even need to condition. Leave conditioners on for at least 5 minutes after shampooing, then rinse out.

quickie conditioner

FOR ALL HAIR TYPES

Add 20 drops of essential oils to suit your hair type (page 163) to 5 tablespoons of a herbal conditioner base from a health food shop.

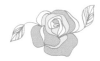

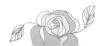

conditioning treatments & masks

hot oil & ginger hair restorer

FOR DAMAGED HAIR

Women have used natural oils as conditioners for centuries. This simple recipe restores damaged hair and eradicates dandruff. Warming the oil before use helps it better penetrate the hair shaft.

3 tablespoons cold-pressed olive oil
2 teaspoons ginger root juice

1   Heat the olive oil in a bain-marie, stirring until warm.
2   Remove from the heat, add the ginger root juice and whisk rapidly.
3   Massage through the hair and scalp then cover with a wet, hot towel for 1 hour.
    Rinse in warm water or diluted apple cider vinegar. Finish with a cold rinse.

egg masks

FOR OILY OR DRY HAIR

For oily hair mix 2 egg whites with 1 tablespoon brewer's yeast. For dry hair mix 2 egg yolks with 1 tablespoon olive oil.

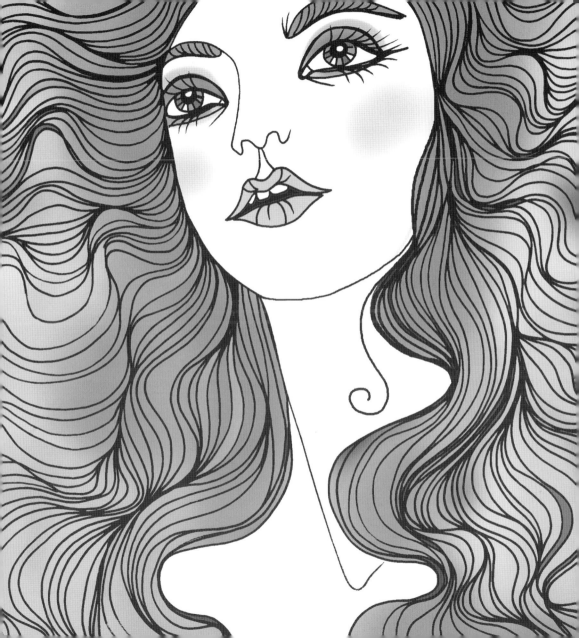

banana & lime hair treatment

This is a delicious and nourishing treat. Coconut oil has been used over the ages as a skin and hair polish. Banana is hydrating and moisturising, and will also add a brilliant shine.

1 egg yolk, beaten
½ banana
2 teaspoons powdered milk
1 teaspoon coconut oil
1 teaspoon lime juice

1 Combine the ingredients in a food processor.
2 Massage through clean, damp hair, leave for 20 minutes, then rinse.
3 Shampoo and condition.

anti-cling avocado hair mask

FOR DRY HAIR

Sleeping on the finest silk pillow slips and patting your freshly washed and dried tresses with a few drops of jojoba oil will help tame frizziness, as will this great mask.

½ avocado
2 tablespoons natural yoghurt
1 tablespoon olive oil

1 Mash the avocado into the combined oil and yoghurt to form a creamy paste.
2 Massage into the hair, leave for 10 minutes, then rinse thoroughly.
3 Shampoo and condition.

rum & egg yolk hair shine

FOR ALL TYPES

Apply this luxurious treatment for shining hair.

2 egg yolks
125 ml rum

1 Beat the egg yolks into the rum.
2 Apply to wet hair, leave for 20 minutes, then rinse thoroughly.
3 Shampoo and condition.

rinses

Rinses can be made from vinegars, or herbal vinegars, infusions and decoctions. They are effective in balancing and healing both the scalp and the hair. A cool rinse can also help close the hair cuticles, resulting in greater shine.

parsley & peppermint rinse

FOR ALL HAIR TYPES

A strong infusion of parsley will help heal the scalp while stimulating the hair and helping to balance the sebaceous glands. It also helps control fly-aways. If your hair is very greasy, add 1 tablespoon of lemon juice.

125 ml peppermint infusion
125 ml parsley infusion

Combine the infusions.

vinegar rinses

Apple cider vinegar makes an excellent rinse, especially if you suffer from a flaky dry scalp. It helps re-establish the acid pH of your scalp and minimise the build-up of hair products and debris. It also helps close the cuticles along the hair shaft, leaving hair smooth and manage- able and helping with fly-aways. Don't worry, the strong fermented scent of the vinegar will not stay in your hair if rinsed well and followed by conditioner.

148

Add 1 tablespoon of apple cider vinegar to a glass of tepid water, pour it over your hair after shampooing and massage into the scalp before rinsing. Alternatively, add 1 tablespoon of a herbal vinegar to 1 cup of water, massage into your scalp and pour through your hair. Finish with a rinse of cold water or herbal infusion. Burdock root, chamomile, dried nettle, horsetail, lavender, peppermint, rosemary, sage and thyme are all stimulating and restorative herbs for the hair and scalp. Use herbs to suit your hair colour (see page 151).

infusion treatments

Herbal infusions, decoctions and vinegars make great final rinses that add shine and lustre to your hair.

hair-styling aids

Hair sprays often contain plastics and other synthetic chemicals that you probably shouldn't breathe in or apply to your hair and scalp. Fortunately, there are some impressive homemade alternatives that work wonders.

detangling spray

Rosemary oil is a blessing when your hair is an unruly tangle. It is essential to shake the bottle before each use, to disperse the rosemary oil throughout the mix.

4 drops rosemary essential oil (or chamomile for blonde hair)
10 drops lavender essential oil
5 tablespoons aloe vera juice
1 teaspoon vegetable glycerine

149

1   Add all the ingredients together in a bottle.
2   This will last up to 3 months in the fridge. Shake before use.

lime & coconut hair wax

FOR ALL HAIR TYPES

This fabulous hair balm will help control and add shine to short hair. Coconut oil is renowned for its restorative properties and has been used for centuries as a skin and hair polish.

15 g beeswax
3 tablespoons coconut oil
2 tablespoons olive oil
20 drops lime essential oil

1   Melt the beeswax and cocoa butter in a bain-marie, mixing well to combine.
2   Remove from heat for a few minutes, then add the essential oils.
3   Pour into a small jar then allow to solidify at room temperature. Store in the fridge.

colorants

Colouring hair with natural products will not yield results as dramatic as those produced by synthetic dyes. The advantage is that you are not exposing yourself to harmful chemicals and that the condition of your hair will be greatly improved. Natural colour enhancers will add shine and colour accents to your tresses, while boosting the health of your hair and scalp – just as nature intended. Each person's hair will take a dye differently, so it is important to do a strand test before application.

Avoid using tap water unless it is filtered. The chemicals in untreated water may react with the natural ingredients in the dye mix, sometimes with disastrous results.

black tea, sage & rosemary rinse or paste

FOR DARK HAIR

1 litre water
3 tablespoons dried sage leaves
3 tablespoons dried rosemary
1 tablespoon apple cider vinegar
3 teaspoons black tea
clear henna, to mix (optional)

1 Combine the water, herbs, vinegar and tea in a saucepan and simmer for 30 minutes. Strain. Add enough henna to form a paste, if desired.
2 Massage the mixture into the hair, then cover with a plastic cap or cling wrap and a warmed towel for 30 minutes. Rinse and shampoo as normal.

colour enhancers

Make a big batch using the recipe below and freeze the leftovers for later applications. When using non-herbal ingredients like cranberry juice, go straight to step 3. Do an allergy test on your skin by applying a little of the mix to your arm. Leave for a couple of minutes, remove, then wait 24 hours to see if there is a reaction.

for red highlights in brown hair alkanet root, cranberry juice, red hibiscus petals, red wine, rosehip tea

for strawberry blondes Use the cooled pinkish water from boiled beetroots as a spritzer while sitting in the sun.

for lightening blonde hair and highlighting mousy hair calendula petals, chamomile flowers, ginger root, ground turmeric, rhubarb root and stem, safflower flowers

for covering grey hair (requires a few applications) black tea leaves, espresso coffee, green outer under-ripe walnut husks, sage leaves

for darkening brown hair and adding shine black tea leaves, espresso coffee, parsley, rosemary, sage leaves, walnut husks

for close to black indigo leaves

1 Place ½ cup finely chopped fresh herbs or ¼ cup dried herbs with 1 teaspoon apple cider vinegar and 1 cup boiling water in a non-aluminium saucepan. Cover with a lid and simmer gently until the colour of the liquid is strong.

2 Leave overnight and strain. Repeat the process if a more intense colour is desired.

3 Add a pinch of salt and 1 teaspoon of glycerine to the cup of liquid and mix well.

4 Add enough clear henna to form a paste.

5 Massage the paste into freshly washed, damp hair. Hold the head over a washbasin containing very hot water and steam for 10 minutes. Cover the head with a plastic cap or cling wrap and a hot towel and leave for 1 hour or longer.

6 Rinse thoroughly with warm water.

red wine & cranberry rinse or paste

2 teaspoons ground coffee

125 ml boiling water

4 tablespoons cranberry juice

1 tablespoon red wine

1 tablespoon olive oil

152   clear henna, to mix (optional)

1 Add the coffee to the water, steep for 20 minutes, then strain through coffee filter paper.

2 Add the remaining ingredients and mix well. Add enough henna to form a paste, if desired.

3 Massage the mixture into the hair and cover with a plastic cap or cling wrap and a warmed
   towel for 30 minutes. Rinse and shampoo as normal.

henna

FOR ALL HAIR TYPES AND COLOURS

Henna is an excellent hair conditioner, preventing split ends and giving a lustrous shine. It is available in all colours for all hair types at most health food shops. It works well on all hair types, although grey may take a few goes to build up depth of colour.

Follow the instructions on the henna packet, but for enhanced results here are a few handy tips. Add an egg to the mix for enhanced conditioning. Yoghurt can also help to prevent the scalp from drying out. If your hair is very dry, add some vegetable oil. Replace the boiling water with a herbal decoction suited to your hair type (page 163). A dash of vinegar will help create an acidic environment and protect the hair. Let the paste stand for a couple of hours before application. Do a strand test before applying to a whole head of hair.

rhubarb, yolk & chamomile blonde-enhancing paste

FOR BLONDE HAIR

Chamomile contains apigenin, which has a lightening effect on the hair. This lovely paste will enhance light brown and blonde shades.

28 g dried chamomile flowers
250 ml boiling purified water
3 sticks rhubarb
250 ml purified water
62 ml lemon juice
clear henna or white clay, to mix

1 Make an infusion of the flowers in the boiling water, strain and cool.
2 Make an infusion of the rhubarb by boiling in the purified water for 15 minutes, then strain.
3 Mix the warm infusions with the lemon juice then combine about ½ a cup of the liquid with enough henna or clay make a smooth paste. You can freeze any leftover liquid for use later.
4 Apply the paste to dry hair using a flat brush, working from the roots to the ends. Cover with a plastic shower cap or cling wrap, then a hot towel, and leave for 30–45 minutes. Rinse thoroughly.

hibiscus delight

FOR BROWN HAIR

Fijian women have long used hibiscus flowers to achieve red highlights on brown hair.

3½ tablespoons dried hibiscus flowers
625 ml water, boiled then cooled for 5 minutes

154

1 Immerse the flowers in the boiled water and steep for 30 minutes.
2 Place over a low heat and simmer for 15 minutes.
3 Remove from the heat, cover and steep for a further 30 minutes.
4 Massage into hair, then cover with a plastic cap or clingfilm and a warmed towel. Leave for at least 25 minutes, depending on the desired shade. Rinse until the water runs clear.

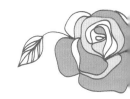
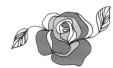
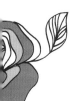
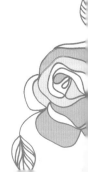
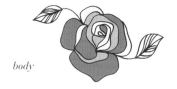

sun care & sunburn

The sun used sensibly is a wonderful beauty aid. It releases feel-good hormones into your system and provides the body with vitamin D, which is essential for healthy, strong bones and teeth. But, like everything, the sun is best in moderation.

natural sunblocks

anti-oxidants Homemade nourishing creams laden with anti-oxidants will also bump up your natural SPF by attacking free radicals on the surface of the skin. To protect the deeper layers of the skin, maintain a diet rich in anti-oxidants like vitamins A, C and E, lycopene, alpha lipoic acid, betacarotene, selenium and co-enzyme Q 10. Foods such as tomatoes, citrus fruits, berries, melons, bright green vegetables, green, black and red tea and goji juice are ideal.

olive oil has been shown to protect skin from future tumours if applied to the skin before UV exposure. Olive oil is high in anti-oxidants, which are probably responsible for this protective effect.

sunblock Look for formulations that use zinc oxide and titanium dioxide. They are both natural sunblocks that offer immediate and effective protection from UVA and UVB rays. For a nourishing natural sunblock, try sesame oil, which has an SPF of 8.

trees Sitting under the canopy of the right tree will protect you from the sun's rays. An oak tree provides an SPF of 10–20, an elm or a sycamore SPF30 and a dense pine forest SPF100.

sundown beauty aids

If you do happen to get burnt, slather these relieving and healing ingredients onto your skin.

aloe vera gel fresh from the leaf or bought at a health food shop.

apple cider vinegar diluted in water.

black tea contains tannic acid that will help remove the heat from sunburn. Apply cool.

milk, buttermilk and yoghurt are all soothing.

oats are very soothing. Wrap in muslin (cheesecloth), soak in warm water and rub over sun-kissed areas.

tomatoes, potatoes, cucumbers or apples Mash or grate the flesh or use the juice.

witch hazel, cool nettle, sage or chamomile tea Freeze wet tea bags and apply them for further relief.

sunburn blister relief

Cornflour, potato flour or rice flour dusted over blisters will dry them and relieve the pain. An added drop of lavender oil will aid healing.

the overly sun-kissed skin spray

This is a wonderfully healing and refreshing tonic for the skin, whether sun-parched or not. Store in a spray bottle in the fridge and it will last you the summer. Spray this over the hair for shine and protection, and to prevent frizziness.

10 drops lavender essential oil
1 teaspoon apple cider vinegar
250 ml aloe vera juice
contents of 2–3 vitamin E capsules

1   Add the essential oil to the vinegar, then mix in the aloe vera and vitamin E.
2   Store in a spray bottle and shake well before use. Keep refrigerated.

sun protection oil

FOR ALL SKIN TYPES

This oil will provide *minimum* protection and is particularly suited to those with darker skin.

125 ml unrefined sesame oil
2 tablespoons calendula infused oil
2 teaspoons vitamin E oil
10 drops lavender essential oil
10 drops mandarin essential oil
5 drops ylang-ylang essential oil

Combine the oils thoroughly.

sun care & sunburn

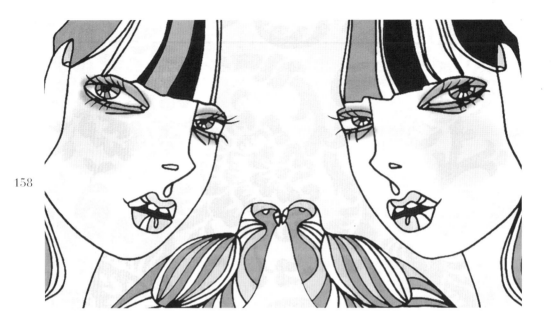

black tea & brush fake tan

During the Second World War, tan stockings were rationed, so women painted their legs with a strong brew of black tea. I use a thick, flat paintbrush to apply this impressive formula. Apply the tea in layers, adding a new one once the last has dried, until you achieve the depth of colour desired.

2 tablespoons black tea leaves
500 ml boiling water

Pour the water over the tea and steep for 30 minutes.

guide to essential oils, herbs, floral waters & foods

skin type or condition

all & normal

essential oils chamomile, geranium, jasmine, lavender, neroli, patchouli, rose, rosewood, ylang-ylang

herbs aloe vera, black tea, calendula, chamomile, comfrey, elderflower, gotu kola, green tea, lavender, licorice root, marshmallow, parsley, rosehip, soapwort

floral waters chamomile, jasmine, lavender, orange blossom, rose

foods almond meal, apple, cucumber, grape, honey, lettuce, melon, oats, papaya (pawpaw), pear, potato, rice, seaweed, wheat germ, yoghurt

milks buttermilk, goat's milk, rice milk, soya milk, yoghurt

oils apricot kernel, grape seed, jojoba, safflower, sunflower, sweet almond

oily

essential oils atlas cedarwood, bergamot, cypress, geranium, juniper, lavender, lemon, lime, mandarin, orange, tangerine, ylang-ylang

herbs alfalfa, aloe vera, bay leaves, burdock root, dandelion, lavender, lemon balm, lemon verbena, raspberry leaves, rosemary, sage, witch hazel, yarrow

floral waters lavender, witch hazel

foods apricots, cabbage, carrot, egg white, grape, grapefruit, honey, lemon, lemon zest, lime, mandarin, orange, papaya (pawpaw), pineapple, strawberry, tomato, watercress, yeast

milks buttermilk, skimmed milk

oils apricot kernel, hazelnut, jojoba, sweet almond

dry

essential oils jasmine, lavender, palmarosa, patchouli, rose, sandalwood

herbs aloe vera, calendula, chamomile, comfrey root, elderflower, licorice root, marshmallow root, parsley

floral water jasmine, rose

foods avocado, banana, carrot, egg yolk, honey, lecithin, melon, papaya (pawpaw), pear, tahini

milks cream, full-fat milk, goat's milk, soya milk

oils avocado, borage seed, macadamia nut, olive, wheat germ

combination

essential oils geranium, lavender, neroli, palmarosa, sandalwood, ylang-ylang

herbs see 'all' and 'oily'

floral waters lavender, orange blossom

foods see 'all' and 'oily'

milks see 'all' and 'oily'

oils apricot kernel, jojoba, sesame, sweet almond

sensitive

essential oils everlasting, German chamomile, jasmine, lavender, neroli, rose, rosewood, sandalwood, yarrow

herbs aloe vera, calendula, chamomile, comfrey, gotu kola, green tea, licorice, marshmallow, red clover, soapwort

floral waters chamomile, orange blossom, rose

foods apple, avocado, banana, honey, melon, oatmeal, papaya (pawpaw), pear, wheat germ

milks buttermilk, goat's milk, soya milk

oils apricot kernel, calendula infused, jojoba, sweet almond

dehydrated

essential oils palmarosa, rose, rosewood, sandalwood

herbs aloe vera, comfrey root, marshmallow root, parsley, rose, slippery elm

floral waters chamomile, orange blossom, rose

foods apple, cucumber, melon, pear

milks full-fat milk, rice milk, soya milk

oils apricot kernel, jojoba, sweet almond

mature

essential oils carrot seed, everlasting, fennel, frankincense, jasmine, lavender, myrrh, patchouli, rose, rosewood, sandalwood, ylang-ylang

herbs elderflower, fennel seed, ginseng, gotu kola, green tea, parsley, rose geranium, sage

floral waters jasmine, rose

foods almond meal, avocado, banana, carrot, egg, honey, orange juice, papaya (pawpaw), peach, tahini, tomato

milks cream, full-fat milk, soya milk

oils avocado, borage, carrot infused, evening primrose, jojoba, macadamia, olive, rosehip, wheat germ

acneous

essential oils bergamot, cedarwood, clary sage, cypress, eucalyptus, everlasting, geranium, German chamomile, grapefruit, juniper, lavender, lemon, myrrh, palmarosa, patchouli, petitgrain, pine, Roman chamomile, tea-tree, thyme, yarrow

herbs aloe vera, burdock root, calendula, chamomile, comfrey, dandelion, echinacea, eucalyptus, garlic, gotu kola, lemon balm, lemongrass, nasturtium flowers, sage, thyme, yarrow

floral waters lavender, witch hazel

foods alfalfa, apricot, cabbage, carrot, grapefruit, lemon juice and zest, lime juice and zest, Manuka honey, plum, strawberry, tomato, turmeric, watercress, yeast

milks rice milk, skimmed milk

oils borage, castor, evening primrose, hazelnut, jojoba

devitalised

essential oils grapefruit, lemongrass, peppermint, rosemary, vetiver

herbs coriander, fennel seed, horsetail, lemongrass, lemon verbena, nettle, parsley, rosemary

floral waters orange blossom, witch hazel

foods bicarbonate of soda (baking soda), citrus fruit, lemon juice, papaya (pawpaw), strawberry, tomato, yeast

dermatitis/eczema

essential oils benzoin, everlasting, German chamomile, lavender, myrrh, palmarosa, patchouli, sandalwood, yarrow, ylang-ylang

herbs aloe vera, burdock root, calendula, chamomile, chickweed, comfrey, dandelion leaf and root, licorice root, marshmallow root, red clover, yarrow

floral waters chamomile, rose

foods cucumber, green beans, papaya (pawpaw), rockmelon (cantaloupe)

oils apricot kernel, borage, evening primrose, jojoba, rosehip

broken capillaries

essential oils blue chamomile, cypress, geranium, lemon, rose

herbs gotu kola, parsley

floral water rose

oil carrot seed infused

body odour

essential oils atlas cedarwood, bergamot, clary sage, cypress, eucalyptus, frankincense, geranium, lavender, may chang, melissa, myrrh, patchouli, pine, rosewood, sandalwood, tea-tree, ylang-ylang

herbs geranium, lavender, lemon balm, lemongrass, lovage, peppermint, rosemary, sage, thyme

scarring

essential oils benzoin, cypress, frankincense, German chamomile, lavender, myrrh, patchouli, rosewood, sandalwood

herbs aloe vera, calendula, comfrey, gotu kola

oils borage, evening primrose, rosehip, vitamin E

warts

essential oils lemon, tea-tree, thyme

hair type or condition

all

essential oils geranium, lavender, rosemary, ylang-ylang

herbs chamomile, henna, horsetail, lavender, rosemary, sage

oily

essential oils bergamot, cedarwood, cypress, geranium, grapefruit, juniper, lemon, lime, patchouli, petitgrain, rosemary, sage, thyme

herbs burdock root, lime flowers, nettle, peppermint, thyme, witch hazel, yarrow

dry & damaged

essential oils frankincense, geranium, lavender, rosewood, sandalwood

herbs aloe vera, chamomile, comfrey, marshmallow root, soapwort

dandruff

essential oils atlas cedarwood, cajeput, clary sage, eucalyptus, rosemary, spike lavender, tea-tree, thyme

herbs horsetail, lavender, nettle, parsley, peppermint, rosemary, sage, thyme

164

children

essential oils German chamomile, lavender, mandarin, Roman chamomile

herbs calendula, chamomile, lavender

inflamed & irritated scalp (with eczema & psoriasis)

essential oils calendula, German chamomile, lavender, patchouli, sandalwood

herbs calendula, chamomile, comfrey, lavender, licorice, marshmallow, parsley, soapwort

hair loss

essential oils atlas cedarwood, clary sage, ginger, lavender, peppermint, rosemary, thyme, ylang-ylang

herbs bay, ginger, horsetail, nettle, peppermint, rosemary, thyme

further reading

Battaglia, Salvatore, *The Complete Guide to Aromatherapy,* International Centre of Holistic Aromatherapy, Brisbane, 2003

Fairley, Josephine, *Organic Beauty,* Dorling Kindersley, Melbourne, 2001

Farrow, Kevin, *Skin Deep: A Guide to Safe, Chemical-free Skincare and Cleaning Products,* Lothian, Melbourne, 2002

Mathews, Megan & Alison Casser, *Radiant Skin, Radiant Health,* ABC Books, Sydney, 2004

Neal's Yard Remedies and Susan Curtis, *Make Your Own Cosmetics,* Aurum Press, London, 1997

Purchon, Nerys, *Bodycraft: Health and Beauty the Natural Way,* Hodder & Stoughton, Sydney, 1993

Rose, Jeanne, *Herbal Body Book,* Grosset & Dunlap, New York, 1976

Stubbin, Carolyn, *Do it Yourself Pure Plant Skin Care,* International Centre of Holistic Aromatherapy, Brisbane, 1999

Tisserand, Robert, *The Art of Aromatherapy,* Daniel, London, 1977

Wildwood, Christine, *Aromatherapy,* Bloomsbury, London, 1996

Worwood, Valerie Ann, *The Fragrant Pharmacy: A Home and Health Care Guide to Aromatherapy and Essential Oils,* Macmillan, London, 1990

Wright, Janet, *Ayurvedic Beauty,* Lorenz Books, London, 2002

suppliers

For a *Feeding Your Skin* starter pack, go to:
www.newdirectionsuk.com/feeding_your_skin

New Directions
Unit 12a Central Trading Estate
Marine Parade, Northam
Southampton SO14 5JP
phone 023 8071 0600

Neal's Yard Remedies
www.nealsyardremedies.com

index

168